COOKBOOK FOR DIABETICS

COOKBOOK FOR

DIABETICS

Compiled by the Ontario Dietetic
Association and the Canadian
Diabetic Association

Revised and Edited for American use
by GAYNOR MADDOX

TAPLINGER PUBLISHING CO., INC.
29 East Tenth Street, New York, N.Y. 10003
1967

PREFACE

All of us who work in the field of carbohydrate metabolism have one great aim — to improve the lot of diabetics everywhere. I am honoured to be invited to write a Preface to this **Cookbook for Diabetics** which has been compiled by the Canadian Diabetic Association in collaboration with The Ontario Dietetic Association. It has been written with great care by a panel of experts and will prove of inestimable value to all who are interested in this disorder. We can be justly proud of the excellence of the material and clarity of presentation.

Charles H. Best, C.B.E., M.D., F.R.S.
Honorary President
The Canadian Diabetic Association

ACKNOWLEDGEMENTS

The authors gratefully acknowledge the contributions made by:

Members of the Canadian Diabetic Association

Members of the Ontario Dietetic Association

Home Economics Section, Canada Department of Fisheries

Consumer Section, Production and Marketing Branch, Canada Department of Agriculture

A special word of thanks is extended to Mrs. A. E. Shields and James Shields, who prepared the final manuscript.

FOREWORD

Cookbook For Diabetics was originally prepared for diabetics in Canada. Not only Canadian readers, however, but also a surprisingly large number of American diabetics found the book valuable to them.

Because of the Canadian edition's unexpected popularity and large sale in the United States, the publishers decided to bring out this new edition adapted to common food terms, market and kitchen measurements, and cooking methods used in the United States. Therefore this edition will have even greater appeal and practicality for Americans.

In this edition, the Cookbook For Diabetics and Exchange Lists For Meal Planning have been bound together in one volume, both adapted by American experts. This one volume edition makes it easier for the diabetic to plan a full eating life than was possible with the two volume edition.

To the millions of diabetics in the United States, this American edition of the trustworthy and highly successful Canadian Cookbook For Diabetics will be welcome news.

Gaynor Maddox
Food and Nutrition Editor,
Newspaper Enterprise Association:

INTRODUCTION

Diabetics, this book is for you! Your meals can be flavorful and attractive, and still conform to your prescribed meal plan. The Cookbook for Diabetics has been compiled to help you prepare and serve appetizing, nutritionally balanced meals and to provide new ideas and culinary inspiration in your daily meal planning.

To make this book possible, a special committee was formed by the Ontario Dietetic Association in 1959 at the request of the Canadian Diabetic Association. Recipes were collected from dietitians and members of the Canadian Diabetic Association. These recipes were then home-tested for palatability, appearance, ease of preparation, and average cost. The final selection of recipes was made to provide popular choices which can add variety to menus, give satisfaction and pleasure in eating, and fit the normal budget allowance of the average diabetic family. In almost every case, the recipe is suitable for family use, so the diabetic may enjoy the same menu as other members of the family. The exchange value, in terms of the Food Exchange Lists in the Meal Planning Booklet, is given for one serving of each recipe. Thus you can see at a glance how it will fit into your diabetic meal plan.

The dietitians who have compiled this book, and the Canadian Diabetic Association which has made possible its publication, sincerely hope that wise and widespread use of the Cookbook for Diabetics will mean more enjoyable meals and better health for more diabetics and their families throughout Canada.

The following members of the Ontario Dietetic Association formed the special Committee to prepare this Cookbook:

Miss Joan Benedict, R.P.Dt.
Miss Edythe Card, R.P.Dt.
Mrs. O. Cikalo, R.P.Dt.
Miss Barbara Hone, R.P.Dt.
Miss Isabel Lockerbie, R.P.Dt.
Mrs. W. Patterson, R.P.Dt.
Miss Corinne Trerice, R.P.Dt.

CONTENTS

All Exchange Lists and values have been converted into terms commonly used in the U.S.A. The *Six Food Exchange Lists* for variety in meal planning published by the U.S. Department of Health, Education and Welfare, Public Health Service was used as the basis for the organization of the recipe material. It is suggested that the reader familiarize himself with these lists which start on page 143.

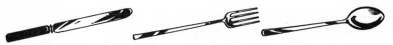

BETTER FOOD PREPARATION

Food should provide both therapy and pleasure for the diabetic. Thus food preparation for diabetics is a serious and exacting responsibility. But it can be made easier and more enjoyable if these facts are kept in mind.

READ THE RECIPE CAREFULLY. The best cooks read through the entire recipe before starting preparation. Then assemble all ingredients and equipment so that preparation can proceed quickly and smoothly.

USE STANDARD MEASURING UTENSILS. Avoid errors and guessing by using a standard eight ounce measuring cup and standard teaspoon and tablespoon. Coffee mugs, tea cups and dessert spoons are not designed for measuring purposes. When measuring fractions, use standard individual measures of 1/4, 1/3, and 1/2 cup, and 1/4 and 1/2 teaspoon.

MEASURE ACCURATELY. Recipes are tested using standard, level measurements. To assure success in using these recipes and to maintain accuracy in diet calculations, make all measurements accurately. Fill the measure and then level it with the edge of a knife or a spatula. Don't guess!

THE OVEN

Term	Temperature (degrees F.)
very slow oven	250 to 275
slow oven	300 to 325
moderate oven	350 to 375
hot oven	400 to 425
very hot oven	450 to 475
extremely hot oven	500 to 525

RECOGNIZE COMMON ABBREVIATIONS.

c. — cup	f.g. — few grains
tbsp. — tablespoon	c.c. — cubic centimetre
tsp. — teaspoon	gm. — gram
oz. — ounce	lb. — pound

1

CHECK EQUIVALENT MEASURES.

1 tablespoon	= 3 teaspoons
1 cup	= 16 tablespoons
⅞ cup	= 1 cup, less 2 tablespoons
¾ cup	= 12 tablespoons
2/3 cup	= 10 tablespoons plus 1 teaspoon
½ cup	= 8 tablespoons
1/3 cup	= 5 tablespoons plus 1 teaspoon
¼ cup	= 4 tablespoons
⅛ cup	= 2 tablespoons
30 grams	= 1 ounce (by weight)
30 cubic centimeters	= 1 fluid ounce
1 teaspoon	= 5 cubic centimeters or 5 grams by weight
1 tablespoon	= 15 cubic centimeters or 15 grams by weight
1 cup	= 8 ounces or 240 grams or 240 cubic centimetres (fluid)
1 Imperial quart	= 5 cups of 8 ounces each (in standard use in Canada)
1 U.S. quart	= 4 cups of 8 ounces each (check this when travelling in the U.S.A.)

REFER TO EXCHANGE LISTS OFTEN. Throughout this book you will find reference to the Exchange Lists. You may need to refer to these Lists often when you try new recipes. Under each recipe, the exchange value of one serving is stated, so that you may easily calculate it as part of the daily meal plan for the diabetic.

YOUR FAMILY CAN ENJOY THESE NEW FOOD IDEAS TOO! The recipes included in this book are not reserved for diabetics only! Often only one family member is a diabetic, and he or she wants to eat the same kinds of foods as others in the group. You will find these recipes suitable for use in family meal planning. From them you can make attractive, appetizing dishes everyone will enjoy. On the other hand, if you live alone or your family is small, you can also use the recipes by dividing the ingredients to make one or two servings. Some slight adjustments in seasonings may be necessary, but these will not affect the food value or calorie value of each serving.

IF YOU USE ARTIFICIAL SWEETENERS: There are several artificial sweeteners, in liquid and tablet form, available for use in food preparation for diabetics. None of these contains any calories, and if used carefully can make prepared dishes, fruits, etc. more enjoyable.

Liquid artificial sweeteners are best for cooking purposes, since they mix easily with other ingredients. If tablets are used, they will dissolve more quickly if crushed first in a spoon. To obtain the sweetening value of 1 teaspoon of sugar, use ⅛ teaspoon liquid artificial sweetener OR one ¼-grain tablet. One word of caution — if foods are oversweetened with artificial sweeteners, they will often develop a bitter flavor. Use too little rather than too much.

If saccharin is the artificial sweetener used, it should be added to the food AFTER cooking. Sucaryl is equivalent to sugar in the following proportions:

1 teaspoon sugar equals 1 tablet or ⅛ teaspoon solution;
one-half cup sugar equals 24 tablets or 1 teaspoon solution.

IF SALT OR SODIUM IS RESTRICTED: Occasionally a diabetic will also be instructed by a physician to restrict salt or sodium in the diet. In this case the salt should be omitted from the recipe, and no extra salt added at the table. The following seasonings and herbs may be safely used to make the food more palatable when salt is restricted. Be careful not to use too much of any of these without experimenting to suit your family's taste:

anise	horseradish (not prepared)	pepper
basil	lemon juice	pimento
caraway	mace	rosemary
chives	marjoram	saccharin
cloves	mint	tarragon
coriander	mustard (not prepared)	thyme
curry	orange peel	
dill	onion juice	
fennel	paprika	
garlic	parsley	

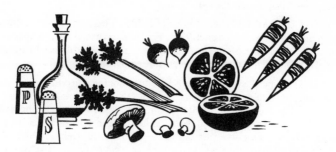

RELISHES AND APPETIZERS

Most diabetics don't need anything to sharpen their appetites at meal time. But they do enjoy a party as much as anyone. If you are planning to serve relishes and snacks to diabetics at your next party, here are some suggestions.

Low Calorie Nibblers

If eaten in reasonably small amounts, as served on a relish tray, the following vegetables make attractive snack foods for the diabetic. In such amounts these could be counted as Calorie Poor Foods List B: celery curls, hearts or small sticks; carrot sticks or curls; flowerlets of raw cauliflower; small green onions or scallions; radish roses or thin slices of white icicle radishes; small Italian or cherry tomatoes; cucumber spears or thin slices; green and red sweet pepper slices or rings; mushrooms.

Canapes and Hors D'Oeuvres

A number of attractive canapes and hors d'oeuvres may be fitted into the day's food allowance. Remember that crackers, bread or melba toast used to carry the fillings must be counted as outlined in the Bread Exchange List.

Here are three delicious fillings which may be spread on crackers or small rounds of dry toast:

LIVER PATE

Yield: 10-12 servings
Exchange 1 tablespoon for: ½ Meat Exchange
Ingredients: 1 lb. calves or beef liver
　　　　　　　　1 medium onion
　　　　　　　　1 large stalk celery
　　　　　　　　2 tbsps. lemon juice
　　　　　　　　salt and pepper to taste

Method: 1. Boil liver in water until tender.
  2. Remove skin, fibre and tubes.
  3. Grind in food chopper with onion and celery.
  4. Blend with lemon juice until smooth.
  5. Add salt and pepper to taste.
  6. Form into a large mound and chill thoroughly.

TANGY LIVER PASTE

Yield: 1½ cups
Exchange 1½ tbsps. for: ½ Meat Exchange
and 1 Foods as desired

Ingredients: ½ lb. beef liver
2 tbsps. chili sauce
1 tbsp. prepared mustard
1 tbsp. mayonnaise
2 tbsps. water
1 small clove garlic (optional)
½ tsp. salt
½ tsp. rosemary

Method: 1. Cook liver in boiling salted water until tender.
  2. Remove skin, fibre and tubes.
  3. Grind in food chopper, using fine blade. Add chili sauce, mustard, mayonnaise, water, garlic, salt and rosemary, and put through the chopper a second time.
  4. Blend together until smooth.
  5. Form into a mound and chill thoroughly.

DILL EGG SPREAD

Yield: 8 servings
Exchange 1 serving for: ½ Meat Exchange
and 1 Fat Exchange

Ingredients: 4 hard cooked eggs
4 tsps. mayonnaise
½ tsp. prepared mustard
¼ cup unsweetened dill pickle slices
1 tbsp. milk
1 tbsp. lemon juice
salt and pepper to taste

Method: 1. Put all ingredients through food chopper.
  2. Blend until smooth.
  3. Garnish with chopped green pepper, chopped pimento or paprika.

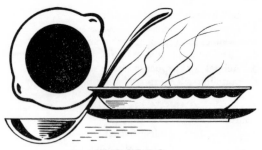

SOUPS

Throughout the ages soup has been one of the most universal of mankind's foods. Today a wide variety of soups is available to add zest and satisfaction to meals. All types of soups may be included in the day's meals for the diabetic, if they are carefully made and if their food values are calculated as indicated in each recipe. Clear soups may be served as an appetizer before dinner. Vegetable soups, with a clear stock base or with a cream sauce base, may serve as part of the main course for lunch or supper. Chowders, thick with fish or meat and vegetables, may be the main course for any meal. For the diabetic who is ill, and whose diet must be restricted to soft or liquid foods, soup can provide ample nourishment in a form that is easy to eat.

The base for many home-made soups is soup stock made from meat, fowl or vegetables. Basic soup stock is a thin, flavorful liquid to which other ingredients may be added to make a variety of soups. Stock soups may be thickened if a heartier soup is desired. If home-made stock is not available, canned consomme or bouillon, or bouillon cubes dissolved in boiling water, may be used in any recipe calling for basic soup stock.

BASIC SOUP STOCK (unflavored)

Yield: 4 cups
Exchange for: 1 Foods used freely
Ingredients: 2 lbs. meat and bone (beef, veal, chicken or mutton)
6 cups cold water
Method: 1. Cut meat into small pieces.
2. Add bones and cold water; soak one hour.
3. Cook below boiling (simmer) for 3 hours.
4. Strain through moistened cheesecloth; save meat if desired.
5. Chill liquid until fat is set.
6. Remove the fat carefully from the broth; discard fat.
7. Refrigerate broth until used.

FLAVORED SOUP STOCK

Yield: 4 cups
Exchange 1 serving for: 1 Foods used freely
Ingredients: 2 lbs. meat and bone (beef, veal, chicken or mutton)
6 cups cold water
1 small onion
½ cup raw carrots, cut into chunks
2 stalks celery, cut into pieces
4 cloves
6 pepper berries
1 bay leaf
1 sprig parsley
1 tsp. salt

Method:
1. Cut meat into small pieces.
2. Add bones and cold water; soak 1 hour.
3. Cook below boiling (simmer) for 2 hours.
4. Add seasonings and vegetables and simmer for 1½ hours longer.
5. Strain through moistened cheesecloth; save meat, if desired.
6. Chill liquid until fat is set.
7. Remove the fat carefully from the broth; discard fat.
8. Refrigerate broth until used.

Unthickened Stock Soups
VEGETABLE SOUP

Yield: 4 servings
Exchange 1 serving for: 1 Vegetable Exchange List 2 B
Ingredients: 3 cups soup stock
¼ cup diced carrots
¼ cup chopped onion
¼ cup shredded cabbage
¼ cup green beans, cut in strips
1 tbsp. celery, finely chopped
2 tbsps. diced turnip
salt, pepper and other seasonings to taste

Method:
1. Add prepared vegetables to the soup stock.
2. Cook until vegetables are tender (about ½ hour).
3. Season to taste. Serve hot.

Note: Any combination of vegetables may be used in this recipe, as long as their exchange value adds up to 1 Vegetable Exchange List 2A, or 2 Vegetable Exchanges List 2B. If you wish to cook the vegetables separately, use only 2 cups soup stock. Add stock to cooked vegetables, reheat and serve.

7

MACARONI SOUP

Yield: 4 servings

Exchange 1 serving for: 1 Vegetable Exchange List 2 B

Ingredients: 2 cups soup stock
½ cup canned tomatoes or tomato juice
½ cup cooked macaroni, drained
2 drops artificial liquid sweetener
seasonings to taste

Method:
1. Heat soup stock and canned tomatoes together.
2. Add cooked macaroni and artificial liquid sweetener. (see page 3)
3. Reheat and season to taste. Serve hot.

Variations:
1. Add 1 tbsp. chopped green pepper, or parsley.
2. Add 1 tbsp. finely chopped celery.
3. Add ¼ tsp. Worcestershire sauce.
4. In place of macaroni, use 1/3 cup cooked rice, noodles or or spaghetti.

ONION SOUP

Yield: 4 servings

Exchange 1 serving for: 1 Vegetable Exchange List 2B
and 1 Fat Exchange

Ingredients: 4 medium onions
4 tsps. butter or margarine
3 cups soup stock
½ tsp. salt
⅛ tsp. celery salt
few grains pepper
1 tsp. Worcestershire sauce

Method:
1. Peel onions; cut into thin slices.
2. Melt butter or margarine; add onion slices and brown lightly.
3. Add soup stock and simmer until onions are tender.
4. Add seasonings and serve hot.

Note: Just before serving, ½ cup grated Parmesan cheese may be added, if desired. If this is done, reheat the soup just until the cheese melts. With cheese, the exchange value of the soup would be:
1 Vegetable Exchange List 2B
and 1 Fat Exchange
and ½ Meat Exchange

TOMATO STOCK SOUP

Yield: 4 servings

Exchange 1 serving for: 1 Foods as desired
1 Vegetable Exchange List 2A

Ingredients: 2 cups flavored soup stock
1 cup canned tomatoes or tomato juice
2 tbsps. sweet green pepper, chopped
2 tbsps. lean cooked ham, chopped
1 tsp. butter or margarine
2 drops artificial liquid sweetener

Method:
1. Combine soup stock and tomatoes and heat slowly.
2. Cook green pepper and ham lightly in butter or margarine.
3. Add green pepper and ham to stock mixture.
4. Add salt and simmer ½ hour.
5. Add artificial sweetener and additional seasonings, if desired.
6. Strain and serve hot.
7. Garnish with chopped parsley or chives.

TOMATO BOUILLON SOUP

Yield: 4 servings

Exchange 1 serving for: 1 Vegetable Exchange List 2B

Ingredients: one 10-oz. can cream of tomato soup, undiluted
one 10-oz. can consomme or bouillon, undiluted
1 cup water

Method:
1. Combine undiluted tomato soup, consomme and water.
2. Heat and season to taste. Serve hot.

Variation: Instead of cream of tomato soup, add 2 cups canned tomato juice to bouillon or consomme. Season, heat and serve. The exchange value for 1 serving would then be:
1 Vegetable Exchange List 2A

Note: The following ingredients may be added to either of these soups without changing their exchange values:
½ tsp. Worcestershire sauce
½ tsp. horseradish
1 tsp. grated onion
1 tbsp. chopped celery
1 tbsp. chopped green pepper

JULIENNE SOUP

Yield: 4 servings

Exchange 1 serving for: 1 Vegetable Exchange List 2B
and 1 Foods as desired

Ingredients: 2 cups flavored soup stock
2 tbsps. cooked carrot, cut in strips
2 tbsps. cooked turnip, cut in strips
1 tbsp. cooked peas
1 tbsp. cooked green or yellow beans, cut in strips
seasonings to taste

Method:
1. Heat soup stock.
2. Add cooked vegetables and reheat.
3. Season to taste and serve hot.

Thickened Stock Soups

CREOLE SOUP

Yield: 6 servings

Exchange 1 serving for: 1 Vegetable Exchange List 2B
and 1 Fat Exchange

Ingredients: 2 tbsps. butter or margarine
1½ tbsps. chopped green pepper
1 tbsp. chopped onion
3 tbsps. flour
2 cups soup stock
1 cup canned tomatoes
2/3 tsp. salt
f.g. pepper
f.g. cayenne pepper
1 tbsp. horseradish
¼ tsp. vinegar
1/3 cup cooked macaroni

Method:
1. Cook green pepper and onion in butter or margarine for about 5 minutes.
2. Add flour slowly, blending thoroughly.
3. Add soup stock and canned tomatoes, stirring to blend thoroughly.
4. Heat, stirring constantly until fully thickened; simmer 15 minutes.
5. Press through a sieve; add seasonings and reheat.
6. Add horseradish, vinegar and macaroni rings. Serve piping hot.

MULLIGATAWNY SOUP

Yield: 6 servings

Exchange 1 serving for: 1 Vegetable Exchange List 2B
and 1 Meat Exchange
and 1 Fat Exchange

Ingredients: 1½ tbsps. butter or margarine
¼ cup each of diced carrots, onions and celery
½ cup diced raw apple, pared
1 cup diced cooked chicken
2½ tbsps. flour
1 clove
¼ tsp. pepper berries
1 sprig parsley
½ tsp. curry powder
2½ cups soup stock
½ cup canned tomatoes
salt, pepper and f.g. cayenne pepper

Method: 1. Cook diced vegetables, apple and chicken in melted fat until lightly browned.
2. Add flour and seasonings and blend thoroughly.
3. Add soup stock and tomatoes and stir over heat until fully thickened; simmer 1 hour.
4. Remove chicken with a perforated spoon or sieve; then press mixture through a sieve.
5. Return chicken to mixture. If liquid has cooked down, make up to 3 cups liquid with boiling water.
6. Reheat and serve hot.

Note: If desired, 3 tbsps. cooked rice per serving may be added to the soup after cooking. The exchange value of one serving then becomes: 2 Vegetable Exchanges List 2B
or 1 Bread Exchange
1 Meat Exchange
and 1 Fat Exchange

Cream Soups

Many milk soups may be made from the same base. This usually consists of vegetable soup stock and pulp, with milk added. Because these soups are usually thickened to the consistency of heavy cream, they are called "Cream Soups". They should be served very hot, and as soon as they are made.

BASIC RECIPE FOR CREAM SOUPS

Yield: 4 servings

Exchange 1 serving for: 1 Vegetable Exchange List 2A or 2B, depending on vegetable or vegetables used, and ½ Milk Exchange

Ingredients: 4 tsps. butter or margarine
3 tbsps. flour
¾ tsp. salt
⅛ tsp. pepper
1½ cups vegetable stock and pulp mixed
1½ cups skim milk or reconstituted nonfat dry milk

Method:
1. Melt butter or margarine, preferably in the top of a double boiler.
2. Blend in flour and seasonings.
3. Add vegetable stock and pulp gradually, stirring until fully thickened; cook until there is no taste of raw starch.
4. Add milk, either hot or cold, and reheat, but do not boil.
5. Serve at once.

Variations of Basic Cream Soup Recipe:

CREAM OF ASPARAGUS SOUP

Exchange 1 serving for: 1 Vegetable Exchange List 2A
and ½ Milk Exchange

Use basic cream soup recipe, adding 1½ cups cooked or canned pureed asparagus plus stock. Add ⅛ tsp. baking soda to asparagus before adding milk, to prevent curdling. A pinch of sage adds a subtle flavor for variety.

CREAM OF CARROT SOUP

Exchange 1 serving for: 1 Vegetable Exchange List 2B
and ½ Milk Exchange

Cook 1½ cups diced, raw carrot and 1 chopped onion in salted boiling water until tender. Press through sieve. Make up to 1½ cups stock plus pulp by adding water. Then follow basic cream soup recipe. Add extra seasoning if desired.

CREAM OF CELERY SOUP

Exchange 1 serving for: 1 Vegetable Exchange List 2A
and ½ Milk Exchange

Cook 1 cup finely diced celery in salted boiling water until tender. Make up to 1½ cups by adding water. Then follow basic cream soup recipe. A teaspoon of grated raw carrot or chopped parsley or f.g. paprika may be sprinkled over the soup at serving time for garnish.

CREAM OF POTATO SOUP

Yield: 4 servings

Exchange 1 serving for: 1 Bread Exchange
and ½ Milk Exchange

Ingredients: 1 small onion, coarsely chopped
1½ cups water
1½ cups skim milk or reconstituted nonfat dry milk
2/3 cup mashed potato
4 tsps. butter or margarine
1½ tbsps. flour
1½ tsps. salt
⅛ tsp. pepper
f.g. cayenne pepper
1 tsp. chopped parsley or grated raw carrot

Method: 1. Cook chopped onion in the water until tender.
2. Add skim milk and reheat.
3. Add this mixture slowly to the mashed potato and blend until smooth.
4. Blend flour and seasonings with the melted butter or margarine.
5. Gradually add potato-milk mixture, stirring constantly until fully thickened; cook until there is no taste of raw starch.
6. If desired, the soup may be strained; reheat and serve at once with chopped parsley or grated carrot garnish.

Note: 1 or 2 tsps. of crushed dried celery leaves, added during cooking, is a tasty addition.

CREAM OF MUSHROOM SOUP

Yield: 4 servings

Exchange 1 serving for: ½ Milk Exchange
and Vegetable Exchange List 2A

Ingredients: ½ cup chopped, canned mushrooms
or ½ lb. fresh mushrooms, peeled and chopped
4 tsps. butter or margarine
3 tbsps. flour
1 cup liquid from canned mushrooms
or 1 cup water
¾ tsp. salt
⅛ tsp. pepper
1½ cups skim milk or reconstituted nonfat dry milk

Method:
1. Cook mushrooms for about 5 minutes in butter or margarine.
2. Mix flour with some of the cold mushroom liquid or cold water, to make a thin paste.
3. Add the remainder of liquid or water to cooked mushrooms.
4. Heat this mixture to boiling.
5. Stir flour paste in slowly, stirring constantly until fully thickened; cook until there is no taste of raw starch.
6. Add milk and seasonings; reheat, but do not boil.
7. Serve at once.

CREAM OF TOMATO SOUP #1

Yield: 4 servings

Exchange 1 serving for: 1 Vegetable Exchange List 2A
and ½ Milk Exchange
and 1 Fat Exchange (page 15)

Ingredients: 2 cups canned tomatoes
⅛ tsp. baking soda
1 tsp. salt
⅛ tsp. pepper
4 tsps. butter or margarine (optional)
2 cups whole milk

Method: 1. Add baking soda and seasonings to cold canned tomatoes.
2. Gradually add cold tomatoes to the cold milk in a saucepan.
3. Heat slowly to serving temperature. DO NOT BOIL.
4. Add butter to hot soup and serve at once.

Note: If butter or margarine is not included, omit the Fat Exchange.

CREAM OF TOMATO SOUP #2

Yield: 4 servings

Exchange 1 serving for: 1 Vegetable Exchange List 2B
and ½ Milk Exchange
and 1 Fat Exchange

Ingredients: 2 cups canned tomatoes
⅛ tsp. baking soda
3 tbsps. flour
1 tsp. salt
⅛ tsp. pepper
4 tsps. butter or margarine
2 cups milk

Method: 1. Heat tomatoes; press through a sieve if desired; add baking soda.
2. Add hot water to make up to two cups liquid plus pulp.
3. In a separate saucepan, melt butter or margarine; blend in flour until smooth.
4. Add milk and seasonings to flour and fat mixture, stirring constantly until fully thickened; cook until there is no taste of raw starch.
5. Gradually add the hot tomatoes to the hot milk sauce, stirring to blend and avoid curdling.
6. Reheat to serving temperature. DO NOT BOIL.
7. Serve at once.

Variations: 1. Add 1 tbsp. finely chopped onion to the tomatoes before heating.
2. Add ¼ bay leaf to tomatoes while they are heating; remove the bay leaf before adding tomatoes to milk sauce.

Note: For the best results when making any type of Cream of Tomato Soup, have the tomatoes and the milk or milk sauce as close to the same temperature as possible. Never allow the mixture to boil.

Special Soups
OYSTER STEW

Yield: 4 servings

Exchange 1 serving for: 2 Meat Exchanges
and ½ Milk Exchange
and 1 Bread Exchange List 4

Ingredients: 2 cups skim milk or reconstituted nonfat dry milk
12 soda crackers (2″ size), crumbled
1 tsp. salt
f.g. pepper
4 tsps. butter
24 oysters plus liquor

Method:
1. Place the first five ingredients in top of double boiler, and heat over boiling water.
2. Drain liquor from oysters, and save liquor.
3. Remove any pieces of shell from oysters.
4. Heat oysters and liquor together slowly until the edges of the oysters begin to curl.
5. Add heated oysters and liquor slowly to hot milk mixture.
6. Reheat to serving temperature. DO NOT BOIL. Serve at once.

CLAM CHOWDER

Yield: 4 servings

Exchange 1 serving for: 2 Meat Exchanges
and 1 Vegetable Exchange List 2B

Ingredients: 1½ cups clams (save clam liquor)
½ cup salt pork, cubed
¼ cup chopped onion
2 stalks celery, chopped
½ cup diced raw potato
2/3 cup water
½ cup canned tomatoes
¾ cup tomato juice
2 tsps. chopped parsley
½ tsp. salt

Method:
1. Chop clams and scald in clam liquor; strain.
2. Fry pork cubes in their own fat until crisp.
3. Add chopped onion and cook until tender.

4. Drain fat from pork and onion.
5. Cook celery and potato in the 2/3 cup water.
6. Add tomatoes, tomato juice, parsley, salt, clams, pork and onion.
7. Simmer 10 to 15 minutes, and serve piping hot. DO NOT BOIL.

CANNED CONDENSED SOUPS

Canned condensed soups may be included in meals for diabetics, if the following exchange values are used:

Exchange: 3 level tbsps. of the soup as it comes from the can for
   either: 1 Vegetable Exchange List 2B
   or: ½ Bread Exchange

For variety, a mixture of two kinds of canned soups may be used. The following liquids may be used to dilute the soup to the desired consistency:

Water: no calories; use as desired

Clear broth, consomme or bouillon: use freely as desired

Milk, skim or whole: Subtract from milk allowance for the meal.

ADDITIONAL SUGGESTIONS FOR SEASONING SOUPS

These may be used for almost any soup, without changing the exchange value of the soup. Use sparingly: whole allspice; ground ginger; thin slices of lemon or lime; chopped parsley; paprika; sesame seed.

For bouillon: celery leaves or celery seed.

For chicken soup : chopped dill; a pinch of marjoram; rosemary leaves.

For consomme: a few cloves; mace; nutmeg; savory ; tarragon.

For fish soups or chowders: basil; bay leaves; curry powder; marjoram; sage; savory; tarragon; watercress.

For oyster stew: mace; nutmeg; thyme.

For vegetable soup: basil; bay leaf; sage; savory ; watercress.

For asparagus soup: chives; sage.

For celery soup: thyme.

For tomato soup: basil; bay leaf; celery leaves; celery seed; curry powder; sage; tarragon.

For soup stock: crushed bay leaf; garlic; ½ tsp. monosodium glutamate.

For tomato, pea or vegetable soup: 1½ tsps. herb vinegar.

For canned soups: ½ tsp. monosodium glutamate.

SOUP ACCOMPANIMENTS

Soup is often more enjoyable with a crisp "bread" accompaniment. Soda biscuits, crackers and melba toast may be served, but they must be calculated as Bread Exchanges. For example, 1 Bread Exchange is equivalent to:

4 rectangular slices or 8 round slices of commercially made melba toast; or one 6-inch piece of matzoh; or 1½ rusks; or six 2-inch soda crackers.

Other soup accompaniments may be made at home:

CROUTONS

Yield: 4 servings

Exchange 1 serving for: ½ Bread Exchange

Ingredients: 2 slices bread, at least 2 days old

Method:
1. Remove crusts and cut bread into ½ inch cubes.
2. Place on baking sheet, and brown lightly in a moderate oven (375°F-400°F).

BREAD STICKS

Yield: 4 servings

Exchange 1 serving for: ½ Bread Exchange
and 1 Fat Exchange

Ingredients: 2 slices bread, at least 2 days old
4 tsps. butter or margarine

Method:
1. Remove crusts from bread slices.
2. Spread each slice with butter or margarine.
3. Cut each into strips, about 1/3" wide and 1½" to 2" long.
4. Place these on a baking sheet and brown in moderate oven (375°F) until crisp.

MELBA TOAST

Yield: 1 serving

Exchange for: ½ Bread Exchange

Ingredients: 1 slice stale bread ¼" thick

Method:
1. Leave the slice of bread whole or cut into four or more pieces.
2. Dry slowly in slow oven (300°F-325°F) until golden brown and crisp.

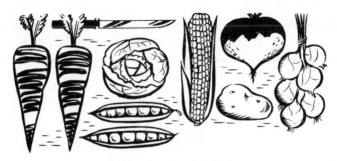

VEGETABLES

Vegetables are an integral part of the diabetic's meal plan. They do not need to be dull, but can be served in an endless variety of interesting ways. The diabetic may eat the same vegetables as the rest of the family, unless salt or sodium must be restricted. In either instance, the diet will be clearly marked: Low Salt OR Low Sodium (see page 3).

The vegetables used may be fresh, frozen, or canned. The size of serving will depend on the type of vegetable used, and the number of vegetable exchanges allowed at the meal.

Most vegetables may be served either raw or cooked. They may be used in salads, soups, and casseroles. Even when served as the vegetable course of the meal they may be cooked in a number of different ways, thus adding infinite variety and interest to such staple fare as carrots, turnips, and peas.

Serving Hints:

Asparagus — serve hot or cold; delicious in salads, either plain or jellied.

Beans, yellow or green — serve hot or cold.

Beets — cook and serve hot with a little vinegar or lemon juice; cook, dice and serve cold in salad; pickle and sweeten to taste with artificial liquid sweetener.

Beet Greens — cook and serve hot; garnish with a wedge of lemon.

Broccoli — cook until tender and serve hot; garnish with a wedge of lemon.

Cabbage — cook and serve hot; in combination with other vegetables in soups or in casserole dishes; serve raw in cold salads.

Carrots — add color to any meal; cook alone or with other vegetables, in a stew, in a number of other meat dishes or in soups; serve raw as carrot sticks or carrot curls, or grated in salads.

Cauliflower — serve raw or cooked. When cooked, may be served hot or cold.

Celery — a very versatile vegetable; raw stalks may be filled with cheese or other filling; chop and add raw to salads; dice and cook in in casserole dishes and soups; boil or braise and serve hot.
In small amounts, (up to 1 tsp. used for flavoring) celery is considered a Free Food.
Note: Celery leaves, dried and crumbled or celery seeds add a piquant flavor to many dishes. Both are Free Foods.

Chard — cook and serve hot; garnish with a wedge of lemon.

Cucumbers — serve raw or cooked.

Dandelion Greens — serve hot as "Beet" Greens or raw in salads. They must be green and tender.

Endive — an interesting and tempting salad green. Wash carefully!

Green Peppers — serve raw in salads, or cooked in casserole dishes and soups; stuff with bread, rice or meat filling or a combination of these and bake.

Mushrooms — serve raw or cooked. Chopped fine and heated with milk and seasonings, they make a delicious soup.
(Don't forget to count the milk!)

Onions — use in small quantities for flavoring meats, casseroles and soups as a Calorie Poor Food; boil, bake, or braise and serve as vegetable course.

Peas — usually served hot; cooked and chilled, they may be added to salads.

Sauerkraut — serve steaming hot with pork chops, pork hocks or wieners; serve cold, if desired.

Spinach — cook and serve hot; garnish with a wedge of lemon; use raw in salads.

Squash — Hubbard, Pepper or Crook-necked — bake, steam or boil and serve hot.

Tomatoes — probably the most versatile and enjoyable of all vegetables; serve hot or cold as outlined in the recipes for vegetables, soups, casseroles and salads.

Tomato Juice — serve hot or cold.

Turnips — dice, cook, mash and season with salt and pepper; if desired, add a drop or two of artificial liquid sweetener when they are being mashed; to add color and flavor as a garnish for salad plates, slice raw turnip very thin and place in cold water to curl.

Turnip Greens — cook and serve hot as the other greens.

The following vegetables have a high starch content. They are considered Bread Exchanges.

Artichokes

Beans, navy or lima, canned or cooked

Beans and Peas, dried

Corn

Parsnips

Potatoes

CREOLE GREEN BEANS

Yield: 4 servings

Exchange 1 serving for: 1 Vegetable Exchange List 2B
and 1 Fat Exchange

Ingredients: 4 strips side bacon
½ medium-sized cooking onion, chopped
2 tbsps. diced celery
2 cups cooked green beans, fresh, canned or frozen.
2 cups canned tomatoes
salt and pepper to taste

Method: 1. Cut bacon into small pieces and fry until crisp.
2. Remove bacon from pan; drain part of the fat from the pan; add the chopped onion and celery to the remaining fat and cook until golden brown.
3. Drain the fat from the onions and celery.
4. Mix the celery and onions with the beans, bacon, and tomatoes in a baking dish.
5. Season to taste with salt and pepper.
6. Bake in slow oven (325°F to 350°F) until the mixture thickens.

GREEN BEANS WITH ALMONDS

Yield: 4 servings

Exchange 1 serving for: 1 Vegetable Exchange List 2A
and 1 Fat Exchange

Ingredients: 2 cups hot cooked green beans

2 tsps. butter or margarine

12 blanched almonds, slivered

Method: 1. Toss butter or margarine and almonds with the cooked green beans.

2. Serve hot.

GREEN BEANS WITH PIMENTO

Yield: 4 servings

Exchange 1 serving for: 1 Vegetable Exchange List 2A

Ingredients: 2 cups hot cooked green beans

1 tbsp. finely chopped pimento

Method: 1. Toss chopped pimento with green beans just before serving.

2. Serve hot.

SPICED BEETS WITH CELERY

Yield: 4 servings

Exchange 1 serving for: $1/2$ Vegetable Exchange List 2B

Ingredients: $1/4$ cup vinegar

1/3 cup water

1 tsp. mixed pickling spice, tied loosely in a cheesecloth bag

$1/4$ tsp. salt

$1 1/4$ cups cooked diced celery

1 cup cooked sliced beets

Method: 1. Bring vinegar, water, spices, and salt to boiling point.

2. Add celery and beets.

3. Reheat to boiling point.

4. Remove spice bag, drain and serve.

HARVARD BEETS

Yield: 4 servings

Exchange 1 serving for: 1 Vegetable Exchange List 2B

Ingredients: 2 cups cooked and drained, fresh or canned beets

$1/4$ tsp. salt

f.g. pepper

$1/2$ tbsp. cornstarch

$1/4$ cup vinegar

1/3 cup water

$1 1/2$ tsps. artificial liquid sweetener

Method: 1. Cut beets in slices or cubes.
2. Mix cornstarch, salt and pepper with cold water and vinegar. Cook until thick, stirring constantly.
3. Add beets and artificial liquid sweetener; let stand ½ hour, keeping the mixture hot until serving time.

CABBAGE

Cabbage may be steamed or boiled until just tender. Do not overcook. It may be served plain, with butter, margarine, chopped cooked bacon or bacon fat, cream, scalloped or au gratin.

CABBAGE SERVED WITH BUTTER, MARGARINE, BACON, OR BACON FAT

Yield: 1 serving
Exchange for: 1 Vegetable Exchange List 2 A
      and 1 Fat Exchange
Allow ½ cup cooked cabbage per serving, and 1 strip crisp bacon crumbled or 1 tsp. butter, margarine, or bacon fat.

CABBAGE AU GRATIN

Yield: 4 servings
Exchange 1 serving for: 1 Vegetable Exchange List 2B
      and ½ Milk Exchange
      and 1 Fat Exchange
Ingredients: 4 tsps. butter or margarine
      2½ tbsps. flour.
      2 cups milk
      ½ tsp. salt
      f.g. pepper
      2 cups drained, cooked cabbage
      4 tbsps. grated cheese
Method: 1. Melt butter or margarine in the top of a double boiler.
2. Add flour and blend until smooth.
3. Gradually add hot milk; stir and cook until there is no taste of raw starch.
4. Add salt, pepper, and cooked cabbage; mix well.
5. Place in baking dish.
6. Sprinkle grated cheese over the cabbage and milk mixture.
7. Bake uncovered in moderate oven (375°F) until the mixture is piping hot and the cheese has melted and started to brown (about 20 minutes).

CELERY CREOLE

Yield: 4 servings

Exchange 1 serving for: 1 Vegetable Exchange List 2 B
and 1 Fat Exchange

Ingredients: 4 strips side bacon
½ medium-sized cooking onion, chopped
½ tbsp. chopped green pepper
2 cups celery, cut in 1½"-2" lengths
2 cups canned tomatoes
salt and pepper to taste

Method:
1. Cut bacon into small pieces.
2. Fry until crisp. Remove from pan to a paper towel.
3. Drain fat from pan; return 4 tsps. fat to pan.
4. Cook chopped onion and green pepper lightly in fat.
5. Combine celery, bacon, onion, and green pepper in baking dish.
6. Add canned tomatoes and seasoning as desired.
7. Bake in moderate oven (350°F to 375°F) until the celery is tender and the mixture has thickened; about 25 minutes.

CREAMED CELERY

Yield: 4 servings

Exchange 1 serving for: 1 Vegetable Exchange List 2B
and ¼ Milk Exchange
and 1 Fat Exchange

Ingredients: 4 tsps. butter or margarine
4 tsps. flour
1 cup milk
salt and pepper to taste
2 cups cooked celery cut in 1"-2" pieces

Method:
1. Melt butter or margarine in top of a double boiler.
2. Add flour and blend until smooth.
3. Gradually add the hot milk, stirring constantly to avoid lumps.
4. Cook over hot water until there is no taste of raw starch, stirring frequently.
5. Add cooked celery and seasonings. Mix well and reheat.

Note: 1 tbsp. grated cheese may be added to the sauce without appreciably changing the food value.

BRAISED CELERY

Yield: 4 servings

Exchange 1 serving for: 1 Vegetable Exchange List 2A
and 1 Fat Exchange

Ingredients: 2 hearts of celery
4 tsps. butter or margarine, melted
salt and pepper to taste
1 cup tomato juice

Method:
1. Wash and cut 2 hearts of celery in half lengthwise, allowing one half celery heart (about 3″ to 4″ in length) for each serving.
2. Place in baking pan.
3. Dribble melted fat and seasonings over the celery.
4. Add tomato juice.
5. Bake in moderate oven (375°F) 45 to 50 minutes, or until tender; baste 2 or 3 times during the cooking. If the liquid cooks away, add water or consomme.

CORN, MEXICAN STYLE

Yield: 4 servings

Exchange 1 serving for: 1 Vegetable Exchange List 2B
and 1 Fat Exchange

Ingredients: 4 tsps. butter or margarine
1 tbsp. chopped red and/or green pepper
1 tsp. chopped onion
½ cup plus 2 tbsps. corn kernels, canned

Method:
1. Cook chopped pepper and onion in the fat until the onion is golden brown.
2. Add the corn and mix well.
3. Reheat and serve.

Note: For a larger serving of corn allow 1¼ cups corn kernels, but keep the other ingredients the same as above.
Exchange 1 serving for: 1 Bread Exchange
and 1 Fat Exchange

CORN PUDDING

Yield: 6 servings

Exchange 1 serving for: 1 Bread Exchange List 4
and $\frac{1}{2}$ Milk Exchange
and 1 Fat Exchange

Ingredients: 2 cups canned corn
$\frac{1}{2}$ tsp. artificial liquid sweetener, if desired
1 tsp. salt
f.g. pepper
2 eggs, slightly beaten
2 tbsps. melted butter or margarine
2 cups hot milk

Method:
1. Add seasonings and artificial liquid sweetener to the corn
2. Add eggs slightly beaten, then melted butter or margarine and milk.
3. Pour into a slightly greased baking dish.
4. Place baking dish in a pan with about 1″ hot water in it.
5. Oven-poach until firm in slow oven (325°F).

BRAISED ONIONS

Yield: 4 servings

Exchange 1 serving for: 1 Vegetable Exchange List 2B
and 1 Fat Exchange
and 1 Vegetable Exchange List 2A

Ingredients: 4 medium-sized onions, peeled
$1\frac{1}{2}$ cups canned tomatoes, or tomato juice
salt and pepper to taste
4 tsps. butter or margarine

Method:
1. Parboil onions about 10 minutes.
2. Drain, reserving $\frac{1}{2}$ cup liquid.
3. Place onions in baking dish. Mix liquid (reserved from cooking the onions) with the canned tomatoes or tomato juice and seasonings.
4. Pour over and around onions.
5. Cut a small hollow in each onion. Put 1 tsp. of butter or margarine in each onion.
6. Bake in moderate oven (350°F to 375°F), basting frequently until the onions are tender; about 30 minutes.

EGG PLANT CREOLE

Yield: 4 servings
Exchange 1 serving for: 1 Vegetable Exchange List 2A
                       and 1 Vegetable Exchange List 2B
Ingredients: 8 slices egg plant (about 4" x 4" x 1" thick)
             1 tbsp. finely chopped onion
             1 tbsp. finely chopped celery
             2 cups canned tomatoes
             salt and pepper to taste
Method: 1. Pare each slice of egg plant and sprinkle with salt.
         2. Lay slice upon slice and place on a plate or in a bowl. Place
            a plate on top for a weight and let stand 1 to 2 hours.
         3. Drain. Cut into cubes if desired, and place in a baking dish.
         4. Add chopped onion, celery and canned tomatoes, and bake
            in moderate oven (350°F to 375°F) until tender; about 30
            minutes.

PEAS

Green peas may be served in many of the same ways as green beans.
The size of serving, however, is smaller due to the higher starch content
of peas.

If you use canned green peas, the size serving for 1 Vegetable Exchange List 2A is 1/4 cup. For fresh green peas, or fresh frozen green
peas, the size serving for 1 Vegetable Exchange List 2A is 1/3 cup.

Keeping this in mind, there are many interesting ways in which green
peas may be served.

Minted Green Peas: A little mint, fresh or dried, added to fresh green
peas or frozen green peas while cooking, is a must in many households.
The mint has no calories.

Green Peas with Pimento: Mix 1/2 tsp. chopped pimento with the serving
of peas allowed. The pimento has negligible carbohydrate.

GREEN PEAS WITH MUSHROOMS

Yield: 1 serving
Exchange for: 1 Vegetable Exchange List 2B
              and 1 Fat Exchange
              and 1 Vegetable Exchange List 2A
Ingredients: 4 mushroom caps, sliced
             1 tsp. butter or margarine
             1/3 cup fresh or frozen green peas, cooked,
             or 1/4 cup canned green peas
Method: 1. Lightly cook the mushrooms in the butter or margarine.
         2. Toss mushrooms and butter or margarine with the hot
            cooked or canned peas.

29

STUFFED GREEN PEPPER #1

Yield: 1 serving

Exchange for: 1 Vegetable Exchange List 2B
and 1 Bread Exchange
and 1 Fat Exchange

Ingredients: 1 small firm green pepper
1 slice bread
1 tsp. butter or margarine
1 tsp. chopped onion
salt, pepper
savory, thyme, sage or poultry seasoning
½ to 1 tbsp. water

Method:
1. Cut stem end from green pepper and wash.
2. Remove seeds and membrane.
3. Crumble bread or cut into small cubes.
4. Cook onion slightly in butter; mix with the bread.
5. Add seasonings and enough water to moisten.
6. Fill the center of the cleaned green pepper with the bread mixture.
7. Stand the green pepper in a small pan with about ½" of water in the bottom of the pan.
8. Bake in moderate oven (350°F) until the green pepper is tender; about 20 minutes.

Note: Instead of partially cooking the onion in the butter or margarine, you could add the uncooked onion to the bread and seasonings. Fill the green pepper with the mixture. Dot the top of the filled green pepper with the butter or margarine.

STUFFED GREEN PEPPER #2

Yield: 1 serving

Exchange for: 1 Vegetable Exchange List 2A
and 1 Bread Exchange

Ingredients: 1 small green pepper
3 level tbsps. cooked and drained rice
1 tsp. chopped onion
1 tsp. chopped celery
salt and pepper
1/3 cup tomato juice

Method: 1. Wash and cut stem end from green pepper, and remove seeds and membrane.

2. Place in pan with ½″ to 1″ water in the bottom.

3. Mix cooked rice, chopped onion, celery, salt, pepper and tomato juice together.

4. Fill green pepper with the rice mixture.

5. Bake in moderate oven (350°F to 375°F), basting frequently until the onions are tender; about 30 minutes.

ESCALLOPED POTATOES

Yield: 1 serving

Exchange 1 serving for: 1 Bread Exchange
and ½ Milk Exchange
and 1 Fat Exchange

Ingredients: 1 small potato, peeled
salt and pepper
½ tsp. chopped onion (optional)
½ cup milk
1 tsp. butter or margarine

Method: 1. Slice peeled potato into thin slices.

2. Place a thin layer (half) of potato slices on bottom of an individual casserole dish.

3. Sprinkle lightly with salt, pepper, and the chopped onion.

4. Cover with remaining potato slices.

5. Sprinkle with salt and pepper.

6. Add the milk.

7. Dot top with butter or margarine.

8. Bake in moderate oven (350°F) until potatoes are tender.

Note: If the fat allowance is very low, use ½ cup skim milk instead of ½ cup whole milk. The exchange would then be:
1 Bread Exchange
and ½ Milk Exchange

POTATO PANCAKES

Yield: 8 pancakes or 4 servings

Exchange 2 pancakes for: 1 Bread Exchange
and 1 Vegetable Exchange List 2B

Ingredients: 4 small potatoes, peeled
1 egg, well beaten
1 tbsp. flour
1 tbsp. chopped onion
salt and pepper to taste

Method: 1. Cook and mash potatoes.
2. Add egg, flour, onion, salt and pepper; mix well.
3. Form into 8 flat cakes.
4. Place on slightly greased baking sheet.
5. Bake in moderate oven (350°F) for 20 to 30 minutes, or until brown.

MASHED POTATO PUDDING

Yield: 6 servings

Exchange 1 serving for: 1 Bread Exchange
and ½ Meat Exchange

Ingredients: 2 cups hot mashed potatoes
salt and pepper to taste
1 tsp. grated or finely chopped onion
1 tbsp. chopped parsley
2 tbsps. butter or margarine
2 tbsps. milk
2 eggs, separated
paprika

Method: 1. To the two cups hot mashed potato, add salt and pepper to taste, onion, parsley, butter or margarine and milk.
2. Beat together well with electric beater or potato masher.
3. Add egg yolks which have been beaten until light and fluffy.
4. Mix thoroughly with the potato mixture.
5. Fold in the stiffly beaten egg whites.
6. Place in a shallow, lightly greased pan; sprinkle with paprika, and bake in moderate oven (350°F) for 30 to 40 minutes, until the potatoes are light golden brown.
7. Serve immediately, cutting into 6 equal portions.

STUFFED BAKED POTATO

Yield: 4 servings

Exchange 1 serving for: 1 Bread Exchange
and 1 Fat Exchange

Ingredients: 4 small potatoes, skins on
salt and pepper
½ tsp. grated onion
4 tsps. butter or margarine
1 egg white, beaten until stiff
paprika

Method:
1. Scrub 4 small potatoes of uniform size.
2. Pierce skins with a fork.
3. Bake until tender in hot oven (400°F to 425°F).
4. Remove from the oven. Slice thin top from each potato, lengthwise.
5. Remove cooked potato from skins, leaving skins intact.
6. Mash potato. Add salt, pepper, grated onion, 2 tsps. butter or margarine and mix well.
7. Fold in stiffly beaten egg white.
8. Pile the potato mixture back into the four potato shells, dividing the mixture equally.
9. Sprinkle with paprika and dot with remaining butter or margarine. Return to oven until thoroughly heated, and slightly browned.

MASHED SQUASH

Yield: 4 servings

Exchange 1 serving for: 1 Vegetable Exchange List 2B
and 1 Fat Exchange

Ingredients: 2 cups hot cooked mashed winter squash
4 tsps. butter or margarine
½ tsp. artificial liquid sweetener, if desired
salt and pepper to taste
¼ tsp. ground cinnamon

Method:
1. To the hot mashed squash, add the other ingredients and mix well.

Note: If desired, a few drops of lemon juice may be added.

SQUASH BAKED OR STEAMED IN THE SHELL

Exchange ½ cup mashed squash for: 1 Vegetable Exchange List 2B
and 1 Fat Exchange

Method: 1. Wash and cut winter squash in halves or quarters
2. Rub 1 tsp. butter or margarine over cut edges of each serving.
3. Sprinkle with salt and pepper.
4. Bake in hot oven (400°F) about 40 minutes or until tender; or steam over boiling water until tender.
5. Remove squash from the shell; mash and season to taste; reheat if necessary.

BAKED TOMATO

Yield: 1 serving

Exchange for: 1 Vegetable Exchange List 2A

Ingredients: 1 medium-sized tomato
salt and pepper
other seasonings to taste, such as a sprinkling of basil, thyme; ½ tsp. chopped onion; chopped parsley; sage or chive

Method: 1. Wash tomato and cut out the stem end.
2. Place in a small baking dish with a little water in the bottom (about ½").
3. Sprinkle with seasonings of choice.
4. Bake in moderate oven (350°F) until tomato is just tender, but not so soft it will fall apart (15 to 20 minutes).

ESCALLOPED TOMATO

Yield: 4 servings

Exchange 1 serving for: 1 Vegetable Exchange List 2B
and 1 Fat Exchange

Ingredients: 1 tsp. chopped onion
4 tsps. butter or margarine
1½ cups canned tomatoes
1 slice bread
salt and pepper to taste

Method: 1. Cook onion slightly in butter or margarine.
2. Add tomatoes, bread cut into small cubes, and salt and pepper.
3. Heat thoroughly.

TOMATOES WITH ONION AND GREEN PEPPER

Yield: 4 servings

Exchange 1 serving for: 1 Vegetable Exchange List 2A

Ingredients: 2 cups canned tomatoes
1 tbsp. chopped green pepper (or celery)
1 tbsp. chopped onion
salt and pepper to taste

Method:
1. Combine tomatoes, green peper and onion.
2. Simmer until green pepper and onion are tender, about 10 to 15 minutes.
3. Season to taste and serve.

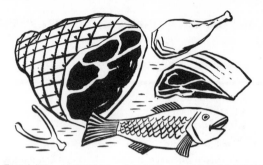

MEAT, FISH AND POULTRY

Dieter's Grace

> Now I sit me down to eat,
> I pray the Lord I will not cheat,
> If I should reach for cake or bread,
> Please guide my hand to meat instead.

Anonymous

Meat, fish and poultry are excellent sources of high quality protein, and are rich in many important minerals and vitamins. These foods are particularly important to the diabetic, since they provide one of the main sources of protein in the meal pattern.

CARE AND HANDLING:

These foods are highly perishable. To preserve both flavor and nutritive values, they should be handled carefully from the time they are purchased until they are served. Because they are particularly susceptible to spoilage and to food poisoning bacteria, meat, fish and poultry should be prepared, cooked and served in sanitary surroundings, and should be protected from contamination and heat during storage.

Always remove the store wrappings from meat and poultry when you return from shopping. Since both meat and poultry tend to absorb other flavors, they should be re-wrapped or covered during storage. For freezer storage, this wrapping should be a moisture-vapor-proof material.

Whether raw or cooked, **meat** and **poultry** should be kept in the coldest part of the refrigerator or in the freezer. It is preferable to thaw frozen meat or poultry before cooking, and if time permits, the thawing should be done in the refrigerator. Once thawed, raw meat or poultry should be cooked as soon as possible. Although raw meat or poultry should not be refrozen, once these foods are cooked, they may be frozen again for further storage.

Fish should be well wrapped or tightly covered if stored in the refrigerator, to protect other foods from fish flavors. Frozen fish may be cooked without pre-thawing, but additional time should be allowed. Once thawed, raw or cooked fish should not be refrozen.

COOKING:

Meat: As a general rule, low temperatures are recommended to reduce shrinkage, improve flavor, retain juices, and produce an even degree of doneness. Dry heat may be used for tender cuts of meat; less tender cuts should be cooked by moist heat. The method of cooking will depend upon the cut and quality of meat purchased.

An oven temperature of 325°F is recommended. For best results, roast meat uncovered and use a meat thermometer. Pierce the meat with a skewer or an ice pick, and push the bulb of the thermometer into the thickest part of the roast, away from bone or fat. (See Roasting Table for times and temperature readings.)

Poultry: As with meats, there are many methods of cooking poultry. Again, low temperatures are recommended to produce tender, moist, flavorful meat, and to reduce shinkage to a minimum.

Except for very small birds, which require slightly higher temperatures, an oven temperature of 325°F is recommended. A meat thermometer is the surest guide to doneness. It should be inserted into the centre of the dressing in a stuffed bird, or into the centre of a thick muscle on the inside of a thigh in an unstuffed bird. Be sure the thermometer does not rest on a bone. (See Roasting Table for times and temperature readings.)

Fish: All fish should be cooked gently, but quickly. Temperatures ranging from 400°F to 450°F are recommended for baking. Most kinds of fish may be baked, broiled, or pan broiled. Fish with stronger flavors may be simmered in moist heat. To test fish for donenes, flake it gently with a fork. If it flakes easily, it is cooked.

COOKING TERMS AND DEFINITIONS

Bake: to cook by dry heat, usually in an oven. This process is called **roasting** when applied to meat.

Barbecue: to roast by direct heat on a spit, over coals, or in an oven broiler, basting frequently with sauce.

Baste: to moisten food during cooking with liquid fat drippings, or other liquid, by ladling the liquid over the food.

Boil: to cook in liquid at boiling temperature (212°F at sea level). The word is sometimes wrongly used to describe "simmering", as in the case of "boiled" eggs or ham.

Braise: to brown meat or vegetables in a small amount of hot fat and then cover and cook slowly, either in the juices, or in a small amount of added liquid, in the oven or on top of the stove.

Broil: to cook by direct heat, under a broiler unit or burner, or over an open fire. Also referred to as **grilling.**

Dredge: to coat with a dry ingredient such as flour or salt, by sprinkling, dipping or rolling.

Fricassee: to cook by braising, often with the addition of a sauce.

Fry, Pan-Fry: to cook in a small amount of hot fat or oil in a shallow pan. Sometimes referred to as **sauteing.**

Grill: see **broil.**

Marinate: to let stand in a liquid, usually an oil and acid mixture such as French dressing, until seasoned.

Pan-Broil: to cook uncovered, in a hot shallow pan ungreased or lightly greased, pouring off fat as it accumulates.

Poach: to cook gently in liquid at simmering temperature (just below boiling) so that food retains its shape.

Oven Poach: to bake, with baking pan placed in a shallow pan of water to slow the baking process and avoid curdling.

Roast: see **bake.**

Saute: see **pan-fry.**

Sear: to brown the surface of meat by short application of intense heat, to improve appearance, develop flavor and seal in juices.

Simmer: to cook in liquid just below boiling point; the surface of the liquid should barely ripple.

Steam: to cook covered, directly over boiling water, or in a tightly covered utensil in which steam is circulating.

Stew: to simmer or boil in a small quantity of liquid. For meats, simmering temperature is always used.

ROASTING TABLE FOR MEATS AND POULTRY

Food	Description	Oven Temp.	Minutes per lb.	Interior Thermometer Reading
Beef	rare	325°F	20 to 30	130°F to 140°F
	medium	325°F	25 to 35	140°F to 150°F
	well done	325°F	30 to 40	150°F to 170°F
Lamb	leg with bone	325°F	25 to 30	180°F
	shoulder, rolled	325°F	35 to 40	180°F
Pork	loin, centre cut	325°F	35 to 45	185°F
	shoulder, rolled	325°F	55 to 60	185°F
Veal	leg	325°F	35 to 45	180°F
	shoulder, rolled	325°F	50 to 55	180°F
Duck		325°F	30 to 35	190°F (in meat)
Chicken	roasting	325°F	30 to 45	165°F (in stuffing) 190°F (in thigh)
Turkey	8 to 10 lbs.	325°F	30 to 35	for all weights,
	10 to 16 lbs.	325°F	28 to 30	160°F (in stuffing)
	18 to 25 lbs.	325°F	25 to 28	190°F (in thigh)

Note: The number of minutes per pound indicated for each food is merely a guide. The surest test that your meat or poultry has reached the desired degree of doneness is by using a meat thermometer. The interior thermometer readings given in the table indicate well done meat or poultry unless otherwise noted.

HERBS AND SEASONINGS

A variety of herbs and seasonings can vary the flavor of meats, poultry, fish and other dishes in a most delicious sense. Don't be afraid to experiment with your favorite combinations of herbs and spices. Keep the following tips in mind:

— Purchase in small amounts and keep in tightly covered containers.

— Test for freshness from time to time, especially those not used often.

— Use sparingly. Excessive amounts will mask the flavor of the food you are trying to improve.

— Add seasonings and herbs during latter part of cooking time, to improve flavor and develop aroma.

— Tie mixed herbs and seasonings in a small cheesecloth bag, so they may be removed easily after cooking.

— Choose one predominate flavor, and blend others with it.

— Monosodium glutamate (M.S.G.) will enhance the flavor of any meat dish. Use about 1 teaspoon per pound of meat, during cooking.

The following suggestions will help you to season your foods expertly:

With Roast Beef: basil; coriander; rosemary; bay leaf; dill; thyme; horseradish; mustard.

With Beef and Veal Stews: bay leaf; thyme; sage; parsley; garlic; marjoram; summer savory; grated lemon rind; celery seed.

With Boiled Beef: horseradish; thyme; cloves.

With Pork: caraway; sage; basil; savory; fennel.

With Ham: nutmeg; mace; coriander; cinnamon; cloves; mustard.

With Liver: basil; thyme.

With Chicken: lemon, paprika; orange; thyme; chives; rosemary; chervil; bay leaf; parsley; celery; caraway; marjoram.

With Fish: anise (shellfish); celery; capers; green pepper; lemon.

Note: Many herbs and seasonings are sold powdered or salted. Herb salts and monosodium glutamate must be omitted from foods for diets restricted in salt or sodium.

SPICED POT ROAST

Yield: 8 servings

Exchange one 3-oz. serving or 3 slices each measuring 4" x 2" x 1/4" for: 3 Meat Exchanges

Ingredients: 2 lbs. boneless chuck beef
1 medium onion, sliced
1 bay leaf
salt, pepper, vinegar, water
1 tsp. whole pepper berries

Method: 1. Rub meat with salt and pepper and place in a china or glass bowl.
2. Add onion, bay leaf, and whole pepper berries.
3. Marinate meat in equal parts of vinegar and water for 24 hours. Drain and reserve liquid.
4. Place meat in roasting pan; sear well; add 3 tbsps. spiced vinegar mixture.
5. Cover and cook in slow oven (325°F) for 1½ hours.

SWISS STEAK

Yield: 4 servings

Exchange 1 serving for: 3 Meat Exchanges

Ingredients: 1 lb. round steak
2 medium onions, sliced
2 tsps. vinegar
½ cup celery, diced
seasonings to taste

Method: 1. Trim round steak and portion into 4 equal servings. Pound to break down tissue.
2. Sear meat on both sides.
3. Cover with water; add vinegar, onion, celery, and seasonings.
4. Continue cooking in oven or on stove until tender.

Variation: 2 cups tomato juice may be used in place of water.

BEEF STEW

Yield: 4 servings

Exchange 1 serving for: 3 Meat Exchanges
and 1 Vegetable Exchange List 2B
and 1 Bread Exchange

Ingredients: 1 lb. lean cubed beef
¼ cup sliced onions
2 bay leaves
6 small whole carrots
4 small potatoes, peeled

Method: 1. Cube beef in 1½″ cubes; sear on all sides.
2. Cover meat with boiling water; add onions and bay leaves
Cover pot and simmer for 1½ hours.
3. Add vegetables and cook ½ hour longer.

HAMBURGER

Yield: 1 hamburger

Exchange for: 3 Meat Exchanges

Ingredients: 9 tbsps. lean ground beef (½ cup + 1 tbsp.)
grated onion to taste
seasonings; such as salt, pepper, sage, thyme, and garlic salt
to taste

Method: 1. Add seasonings and onion to meat and form into 1 patty.
2. Broil or fry in part of fat allowance. If cooking on top of
stove, add a little water when meat is seared to avoid
sticking.

HAMBURGER STUFFED TOMATOES

Yield: 4 servings

Exchange 1 serving for: 2 Meat Exchanges
and 1 Vegetable Exchange List 2B

Ingredients: 4 medium-sized tomatoes
¾ lb. lean ground beef
1 tbsp. grated onion
1 tbsp. chopped parsley
1 tsp. Worcestershire sauce
salt and pepper to taste
¼ cup bread crumbs
¼ cup grated cheese

Method: 1. Remove stem ends of tomatoes; scoop out some of the pulp and drain tomatoes.
2. Combine beef, tomato pulp, and seasonings and stuff tomato shells with the mixture, dividing it evenly.
3. Sprinkle with mixture of bread crumbs and grated cheese.
4. Place in baking dish and bake in moderate oven (375°F) for 30 minutes.

MEAT LOAF #1

Yield: 4 servings

Exchange 1 serving for: 3 Meat Exchanges

Ingredients: 1 lb. lean ground beef
1 egg, slightly beaten
1 tbsp. chopped onion
½ tsp. salt
¼ tsp. pepper

Method: 1. Mix ingredients and mold into a loaf pan.
2. Bake in moderate oven (375°F) for 30 to 45 minutes.

MEAT LOAF #2

Yield: 4 servings

Exchange 1 serving for: 3 Meat Exchanges
and 1 Vegetable Exchange List 2B

Ingredients: 1 lb. lean ground beef
2 tbsps. minced green pepper
1 tbsp. chopped onion
1½ cups tomato juice
¼ tsp. Worcestershire sauce
½ tsp. artificial liquid sweetener
½ tsp. salt
¼ tsp. pepper

Method: 1. Mix ingredients and mold into a loaf pan.
2. Bake in moderate oven (375°F) for 30 to 45 minutes.

BEEF PORCUPINES

Yield: 4 servings

Exchange 1 serving for: 3 Meat Exchanges
and 1 Vegetable Exchange List 2 B
and 1 Bread Exchange

Ingredients: 1 lb. lean ground beef chuck
1 tsp. baking powder
1 medium-sized onion, grated
1 tbsp. chopped parsley
1/3 cup skim milk or reconstituted nonfat dry milk
1 tsp. salt
1/4 tsp. black pepper
1/3 cup washed, drained, uncooked rice
1/4 tsp. thyme
1/8 tsp. cloves
1/8 tsp. poultry seasoning
1 tsp. Worcestershire sauce
half 10 oz. can tomato soup, undiluted
3/4 cup water

Method: 1. Mix all ingredients except soup and water. Form into patties and place in baking dish.
2. Mix soup and water and pour over patties.
3. Bake uncovered, in a moderate oven (350°F) for 35 minutes. Cover and continue baking for 30 minutes.

BAKED HAM SLICE — MUSTARD SAUCE

Yield: 4 servings

Exchange 1 serving for: 3 Meat Exchanges
and 1/2 Fruit Exchange List 3

Ingredients: 1 lb. ham slice, about 1″ thick
1/2 tsp. artificial liquid sweetener
1/4 tsp. mustard
1/4 tsp. Worcestershire sauce
2 tbsps. water
1/2 cup unsweetened pineapple juice
pinch of salt
pinch of paprika

Method: 1. Blend seasonings with pineapple juice and water and pour over ham slice.
2. Bake in moderate oven (350°F) for 20 to 30 minutes.

NEW ENGLAND BOILED DINNER (one-dish meal)

Yield: 8 servings

Exchange 1 serving for: 3 Meat Exchanges
and 1 Vegetable Exchange List 2A
and 1 Vegetable Exchange List 2B
and ½ Bread Exchange

Ingredients: 2 lbs. lean corned beef or boiling beef
4 whole small carrots
1 cup diced turnip
4 small potatoes, peeled
4 wedges cabbage
4 small onions
salt and pepper to taste

Method: 1. Cover beef with cold water and bring to a boil.
2. Simmer in tightly covered pan for one hour.
3. Add all vegetables except cabbage and simmer ½ hour longer.
4. Add cabbage and cook uncovered for 15 minutes.

BROILED HAM PATTIES

Yield: 4 servings

Exchange 1 serving for: 2 Meat Exchanges
and ½ Fruit Exchange

Ingredients: 1 egg
2 cups ground cooked ham
1 tsp. chopped onion
seasonings to taste
4 slices unsweetened canned pineapple
4 tbsps. unsweetened pineapple juice

Method: 1. Add beaten egg to minced ham and chopped onion.
2. Season to taste.
3. Form into 4 patties of equal size.
4. Halve the pineapple slices; place four halves on baking sheet; top each with ham patty. Place remaining pineapple slices on top of ham patties.
5. Pour the pineapple juice over patties.
6. Bake in moderate oven at (350°F) for 15 minutes.

BACON BURGERS

Yield: 4 servings

Exchange 1 serving for: 3 Meat Exchanges
and 1 Fat Exchange

Ingredients: 4 strips bacon
¾ lb. lean ground beef
¼ lb. lean ground pork
1 tbsp. chopped parsley
1 tbsp. chopped onion
⅛ tsp. each of thyme, mace, sage, savory
1 tbsp. green pepper, chopped
¾ tsp. salt
¼ tsp. pepper

Method: 1. Combine all ingredients, except bacon.
2. Shape into 4 patties.
3. Broil 5 minutes on each side and continue cooking to desired degree of doneness. Broil bacon at the same time.
4. Garnish meat patties with crisp bacon slices.

SPARERIBS

Yield: 4 servings

Exchange 1 serving for: 3 Meat Exchanges
and 1 Vegetable Exchange List 2A

Ingredients: 2 lbs. pork spareribs, cut in pieces
1 lemon, sliced
1 onion, sliced
½ cup catsup
1/3 cup Worcestershire sauce
1 tsp. chili powder
1 tsp. salt
2 dashes Tabasco
2 cups water

Method: 1. Place ribs in shallow pan; top with lemon slice and onion slice; secure with a toothpick.
2. Roast in a very hot oven (450°F) for ½ hour.
3. Heat remaining ingredients to boiling point and pour over spareribs.
4. Bake in moderate oven (350°F) for 1 hour, basting every 15 minutes.

VEAL SCALLOPINI

Yield: 4 servings

Exchange 1 serving for: 3 Meat Exchanges
and 1 Vegetable Exchange List 2B

Ingredients: 1 lb. stewing veal, cut in 2″ cubes
½ cup thinly sliced onions
½ cup thinly sliced carrots
1 lb. thinly sliced mushrooms
¼ tsp. paprika
1¼ cups water
2 tsps. shortening or margarine
salt and pepper
juice of 1 lemon

Method: 1. Pan-fry diced veal in shortening or margarine.
2. Add vegetables, seasonings, water and simmer until tender.
3. Add more water gradually as liquid simmers down.
4. Just before serving, add lemon juice.
5. Serve with cooked noodles.

Note: Allow 1/3 cup cooked noodles for 1 Bread Exchange.

BARBECUED CHICKEN

Yield: 4 servings

Exchange 1 serving for: 3 Meat Exchanges
and 1 Vegetable Exchange List 2A

Ingredients: one 2 lb. broiler-fryer chicken
¼ cup vinegar
½ cup catsup
dash of Tabasco
1 cup water

Method: 1. Cut chicken into serving portions and place in a baking pan, skin side down.
2. Mix other ingredients and pour over chicken.
3. Bake in moderate oven (350°F) for ½ hour.
4. Turn chicken over, baste with sauce and continue baking for another half hour.

LEMON BARBECUED CHICKEN

Yield: 4 servings

Exchange 1 serving for: 3 Meat Exchanges
and 1 Fat Exchange

Ingredients: one 2 lb. broiler-fryer chicken
¼ cup lemon juice
⅛ cup melted butter or margarine
1 small onion, grated
1 clove garlic, minced
½ tsp. salt
½ tsp. celery salt
½ tsp. black pepper
½ tsp. rosemary
¼ tsp. thyme

Method: 1. Cut chicken into serving portions and marinate in barbecue mixture (made by combining remaining ingredients) for several hours.
2. Broil chicken pieces, turning and brushing often with marinade, until done.

CHICKEN CHOP SUEY

Yield: 4 servings

Exchange 1 serving for: 3 Meat Exchanges
and 1 Vegetable Exchange List 2B

Ingredients: ½ cup mushrooms
one 2 lb. broiler-fryer chicken
½ cup chopped green pepper
1 cup diced celery
½ cup chopped onion
1 cup bean sprouts
2 tbsps. flour
2 tbsps. soy sauce

Method: 1. Simmer chicken in water until meat will fall from bones.
2. Separate meat and broth.
3. Cook celery, onion, and pepper slowly in ½ cup of chicken broth.
4. Add shredded chicken and bean sprouts.
5. Thicken remaining chicken broth by making a paste with flour. Add to chicken mixture, and stir until thickened.
6. Stir in soy sauce and mushrooms. Serve plain or on rice.

Note: This recipe does not include the rice.
If rice is used, allow 1/3 cup cooked rice for 1 Bread Exchange.

BROILED LIVER

Yield: 1 serving

Exchange for: 3 Meat Exchanges

Ingredients: one 4-oz. portion beef or calves liver, 1/3" thick

Method:
1. Dry liver slices on paper towel.
2. Place liver on broiling rack, 3" from broiler; leave door of oven open slightly.
3. Broil liver on each side. Season with salt and pepper, if desired.

BURGER KABOBS

Yield: 4 servings

Exchange 1 kabob for: 3 Meat Exchanges
and 1 Vegetable Exchange List 2A

Ingredients: 1 large green pepper
4 small onions
1 lb. lean ground beef
¾ tsp. monosodium glutamate
¾ tsp. salt
¼ tsp. pepper

Method:
1. Cut green pepper into 8 large pieces and cut onions in half.
2. Mix lean minced beef and spices and shape into 12 meat balls.
3. Thread on a skewer (3 on each skewer) alternately with green pepper and onion.
4. Cook over barbecue grill, turning often until meat is done.

KABOB OF CHICKEN LIVERS

Yield: 4 kabobs

Exchange 1 kabob for: 3 Meat Exchanges
and 1 Fat Exchange
and 1 Foods as desired

Ingredients: 1 lb. chicken livers
½ lb. mushroom caps
4 tsps. butter or margarine
salt, pepper, onion salt

Method:
1. Alternate chicken livers and mushroom caps on skewer. Brush lightly with butter or margarine.
2. Broil 3" from broiler for 10 minutes, turning often. Season to taste.

FRANK-PINEAPPLE KABOBS

Yield: 4 servings

Exchange 1 serving for: 1 Meat Exchange
and 2 Fat Exchanges
and ½ Fruit Exchange

Ingredients: 4 wieners
4 slices bacon
1 small green pepper
one 8-oz.can pineapple tidbits, unsweetened
4 tsps. salad oil
1 tsp. Worcestershire sauce

Method:
1. Cut each wiener into 3 pieces, and bacon into squares.
2. Cut green pepper into 12 pieces.
3. Alternate pieces of wiener, green pepper, bacon and pineapple tidbits on four skewers.
4. Mix juice from pineapple with salad oil and Worcestershire sauce and brush over kabobs.
5. Broil on barbecue grill for 7 to 12 minutes, turning often.

BAKED HALIBUT ROYALE

Yield: 4 servings

Exchange 1 serving for: 3 Meat Exchanges
and 1 Vegetable Exchange List 2B
and 1 Fat Exchange

Ingredients: 1 lb. halibut steak (boneless)
½ tsp. salt
¼ tsp. paprika
pinch of cayenne
juice of 1 lemon
¼ cup chopped onion
4 tsps. butter or margarine
thin green pepper strips

Method:
1. Sprinkle fish steaks with seasonings and lemon juice.
2. Marinate in refrigerator for 1 hour, turning once.
3. Saute onion in butter.
4. Place steaks in a greased baking dish and spread with sauteed onion.
5. Top with green pepper strips.
6. Bake in hot oven (400°F to 425°F) for 10 minutes, or until fish flakes easily with a fork.

BAKED FISH FILLETS

Yield: 4 servings

Exchange 1 serving for: 3 Meat Exchanges
and ½ Bread Exchange
and 1 Fat Exchange

Ingredients: 1 lb. fish fillets
¼ cup milk
½ tsp. salt
4 tbsps. fine dry bread crumbs
4 tsps. butter or other fat

Method: 1. Cut fillets into four portions and soak 3 minutes in milk, to which salt has been added.
2. Drain and roll in bread crumbs.
3. Place fish on greased baking dish and dot with fat.
4. Bake in very hot oven (450°F to 475°F), allowing 8 minutes if fish is fresh and 15 minutes if fish is frozen, or until fish flakes easily with a fork.

BAKED FISH IN CATSUP SAUCE

Yield: 4 servings

Exchange 1 serving for: 3 Meat Exchanges
and 1 Vegetable Exchange List 2B

Ingredients: 1 lb. fish fillets
2/3 cup chopped onion
1 tsp. butter or other fat
2 tsps. flour
1 bouillon cube, dissolved in ½ cup hot water
4 tbsps. catsup
½ cup sliced dill pickle

Method: 1. Place fish in greased baking dish.
2. Cook onion in fat in a saucepan; stir in flour.
3. Gradually add bouillon mixture and catsup. Cook, stirring constantly until blended.
4. Simmer uncovered for 10 minutes; add dill pickles.
5. Pour sauce over fish.
6. Bake in very hot oven (450°F to 475°F) for 15 minutes (fresh fish) or 25 minutes (frozen fish), or until fish flakes easily with a fork.

51

BAKED FINNAN HADDIE

Yield: 4 servings

Exchange 1 serving for: 3 Meat Exchanges
and 1 Fat Exchange
and $1/4$ Milk Exchange

Ingredients: 1 lb. finnan haddie (smoked fillets of haddock)
1 cup milk
4 tsps. butter or margarine
paprika

Method: 1. Cut fish into 4 servings. Place in greased baking dish; add milk. Dot with butter and sprinkle with paprika.
2. Bake in slow oven (325°F) for $1/2$ hour, or until fish flakes easily with a fork.

FILLETS IN LEMON BUTTER SAUCE

Yield: 4 servings

Exchange 1 serving for: 3 Meat Exchanges
and 1 Fat Exchange

Ingredients: 1 lb. fish fillets
1 tbsp. lemon juice
1 tbsp. finely chopped parsley
4 tsps. melted butter or margarine
$1/4$ tsp. salt
$1/8$ tsp. pepper

Method: 1. Arrange fillets in a greased baking dish.
2. Combine remaining ingredients and pour over fillets.
3. Bake in a very hot oven (450°F to 475°F) for 8 minutes (fresh fish) or 15 minutes (frozen fish), or until fish flakes easily with a fork.

PIQUANT SCALLOPS

Yield: 4 servings

Exchange 1 serving for: 3 Meat Exchanges
and 2 Fat Exchanges
and $1/2$ Bread Exchange

Ingredients: 1 lb. scallops
3 tbsps. fine dry bread crumbs
8 tsps. melted butter or margarine
1 tsp. Worcestershire sauce
2 tsps. lemon juice

Method: 1. Roll scallops in the bread crumbs. Arrange in 4 scallop shells, or in a shallow greased baking dish.
2. Pour mixture of melted butter or margarine, Worcestershire sauce and lemon juice over the scallops.
3. Bake in very hot oven (450°F to 475°F) for 10 minutes.

FISH FILLETS IN MUSHROOM SAUCE

Yield: 4 servings
Exchange 1 serving for: 3 Meat Exchanges
and 1 Fat Exchange
and ½ Bread Exchange
and ½ Milk Exchange
Ingredients: 1 cup fresh mushrooms
3 tbsps. butter or margarine
2½ tbsps. flour
½ tsp. salt
dash of cayenne
2 cups of skim milk or reconstituted nonfat dry milk
1 lb. fish fillets
½ tsp. salt
¼ cup soft bread crumbs
Method: 1. Wash and slice mushrooms.
2. Saute in butter for 5 minutes.
3. Add flour and seasonings, mixing to a smooth paste.
4. Add milk gradually, stirring constantly; cook until thickened.
5. Place fillets in baking dish and sprinkle with salt.
6. Cover with sauce. Top with bread crumbs. Bake in moderately hot oven (375°F) for ½ hour.

CAPER SAUCE FOR FISH

Yield: ½ cup or 4 servings
Exchange 2 tbsps. for: 2 Fat Exchanges
and 1 Foods as desired
Ingredients: 3 tbsps. melted butter or margarine
juice of 1 lemon
1 tbsp. chopped parsley
1 tbsp. minced capers
freshly ground black pepper
salt
Method: 1. Combine ingredients and serve with steamed or boiled fish.

53

VEGETABLE-STUFFED FILLET ROLLS

Yield: 6 rolls

Exchange 2 rolls for: 3 Meat Exchanges
and 1 Vegetable Exchange List 2B

Ingredients: 1 lb. thin fish fillets (sole is especially good)
$\frac{1}{4}$ tsp. salt
$\frac{1}{8}$ tsp. pepper
Vegetable Stuffing:
1 tsp. melted butter or other fat
$\frac{1}{2}$ tbsp. lemon juice
$\frac{1}{8}$ cup chopped onion
$\frac{1}{2}$ cup chopped tomato
$\frac{1}{2}$ cup chopped cucumber

Method:
1. Skin fillets and slice into strips 6" by 2".
2. Season fillets on both sides.
3. Line greased muffin tins or custard cups with fillets.
4. Mix stuffing ingredients together. Season and fill centre of fillet rings.
5. Combine melted fat and lemon juice and pour over rolls.
6. Bake in very hot oven (450°F to 475°F) for 15 minutes.

TO MAKE YOUR OWN SEASONING SALT —

Ingredients: 2 tbsps. salt
2 tbsps. paprika
1 tsp. onion salt
1 tsp. black pepper
$1\frac{1}{2}$ tsps. monosodium glutamate
1 tsp. celery salt
1 tsp. garlic salt

Method:
1. Mix well.
2. Store in tightly capped jar.

CRANBERRY SAUCE

Exchange: 1 tbsp. this cranberry sauce may be taken as a low calorie food and used as desired.

Ingredients: 2 cups raw cranberries
1/3 cup water
1 tsp. artificial liquid sweetener

Method:
1. Cook cranberries and water until very soft.
2. Add artificial liquid sweetener. Chill.

HOT MUSTARD

Exchange: 1 tsp. mustard may be taken as a low calorie food and used freely, if desired.

Ingredients: 3 tbsps. dry mustard
1/3 tsp. artificial liquid sweetener
1 egg, beaten
¼ cup vinegar
¼ cup water

Method: 1. Mix mustard, artificial liquid sweetener, and beaten egg.
2. Add water and vinegar gradually.
3. Cook in double boiler over hot water, stirring constantly until thick.

ORANGE CRANBERRY RELISH

Exchange 1 tbsp. for: ¼ Fruit Exchange List 3

Ingredients: ½ lb. fresh cranberries
1½ oranges
lemon juice
artificial liquid sweetener to taste

Method: 1. Wash cranberries.
2. Wash and quarter unpeeled oranges.
3. Put oranges and cranberries through the food chopper.
4. Add lemon juice and artificial liquid sweetener; mix well.
5. Store in refrigerator for several hours to blend flavors.

TARTAR SAUCE

Yield: 1 cup

Exchange 1 tbsp. for: 1 Fat Exchange

Ingredients: 1 cup commercial mayonnaise
½ tbsp. chopped olives
½ tbsp. chopped pickles, drained
½ tbsp. capers
½ tbsp. chopped parsley
½ tbsp. onion juice

Method: 1. Combine all ingredients and mix well.
2. Serve with fish or veal.

TO MAKE STUFFING FOR WHOLE TURKEY

Yield: Sufficient stuffing for one turkey 10 to 15 lbs.

Exchange ½ cup for: 1 Bread Exchange
and 1 Fat Exchange

Ingredients: 1½ loaves bread (about 34 slices)
2 onions, chopped
2 tsps. salt
pepper to taste
1 to 2 tsps. poultry seasoning
5 tbsps + 2 tsps. melted butter or margarine
water to moisten

Method: Proceed as for individual amount of stuffing.

STUFFING FOR FISH

Yield: 4 servings

Exchange 1 serving for: 1 Bread Exchange
and 1 Fat Exchange

Ingredients: 4 slices bread, cubed or crumbled
2 tsps. chopped onion
2 tsps. finely chopped dietetic sweet mixed pickle
or 2 tsps. capers
4 tsps. melted butter or margarine
water to moisten

Method: Combine all ingredients.

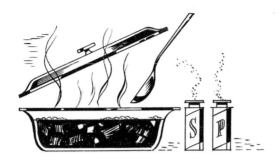

CASSEROLES

Every homemaker dreams of creating memorable dishes from left-overs. A casserole dish is the answer to her dream — and here we offer a collection of recipe ideas so that diabetics and their families may enjoy the subtle blend of flavors and the economy that such dishes afford. Casseroles are helpful too, in preparing meals for the family ahead of time, ready to be served whenever they are needed.

In these recipes, designed with the diabetic in mind, raw minced meat may be replaced with cooked minced or diced meat. Except for ingredients such as eggs or bread crumbs, used as thickening agents, the amounts of the ingredients — meat, vegetables, etc. — may be increased or decreased to suit the amounts allowed in the meal plan of the diabetic.

The recipes are given for family amounts, and any suitable casserole dish may be used for cooking or baking. Individual casseroles are attractive too, and if care is taken in dividing the mixture, the recipe may be baked and served in individual dishes. When baking, place the oven rack so that the top of the product is at the centre of the oven, and place the casserole so it is as near the centre of the oven as possible, for efficient circulation of heat.

SHEPHERD'S PIE

Yield: 4 servings

Exchange 1 serving for: 2 Meat Exchanges
and 1 Bread Exchange

Ingredients: 2 cups ground cooked beef
salt and pepper to taste
1 tbsp. plus 1 tsp. grated onion
1 and 1/3 cups mashed potato
clear fat free broth or consomme

Method:
1. Add seasonings and onion to minced cooked beef. Mix well.
2. Add the broth or consomme to moisten.
3. Place in a casserole dish.
4. Spread mashed potato over the top.
5. Place in moderate oven (350°F-375°F) until heated through and potatoes are slightly browned.

Note: If the Meat Exchange is three for this meal rather than two, use ¾ cup minced cooked beef per serving.

Variations:
1. Pipe potato around edge of casserole dish and garnish with 1 tsp. catsup per serving.
   Increase food value by 1 Vegetable Exchange List 2B.
2. Substitute green pepper (1 tbsp. per serving) for onion.

MEAT VEGETABLE CASSEROLE

Yield: 4 servings

Exchange 1 serving for: 2 Meat Exchanges
and 1 Vegetable Exchange List 2B

Ingredients: 1 cup ground meat
1 cup diced turnip
1 small diced potato
2 cups broth

Method:
1. Cook vegetables in broth 10 minutes; drain, reserving broth.
2. Arrange vegetables in casserole; cover with minced meat; add broth to cover meat.
3. Cover and bake in moderate oven (350°F-375°F) for 1 hour.

MACARONI AND CHEESE #1

Yield: 4 servings

Exchange 1 serving for: 1 Bread Exchange
and 2 Meat Exchanges
and 1 Vegetable Exchange List 2A

Ingredients: 2 cups cooked macaroni
2 cups grated cheese
1 and 1/3 cups tomato juice
salt and pepper to taste

Method: 1. Place cooked macaroni in casserole dish; add tomato juice and seasonings to taste.
2. Sprinkle grated cheese over the mixture and place under broiler or bake in moderate oven (350°F) until cheese is bubbly and browned.

Note: Canned tomatoes may be used in place of tomato juice.

MACARONI AND CHEESE #2

Yield: 4 servings

Exchange 1 serving for: 2 Meat Exchanges
and 1 Bread Exchange
and 1/2 Milk Exchange
and 1 Fat Exchange

Ingredients: 1/2 cup soft bread crumbs
1/4 cup butter or margarine, melted
4 ozs. cheese
2 cups skim milk or reconstituted nonfat dry milk
4 eggs
1/2 tsp. dry mustard
salt and pepper to taste
1 cup cooked macaroni

Method: 1. Toss bread crumbs with melted butter or margarine.
2. Scald milk; add cheese cut into small cubes, and stir until melted.
3. Pour over well beaten eggs; season with dry mustard, salt, and pepper.
4. Add cooked macaroni; cover with buttered bread crumbs.
5. Bake in moderate oven (350°F) for 30 minutes.

MACARONI AND CHEESE #3

Yield: 4 servings

Exchange 1 serving for: 1 Meat Exchange
and 1 Bread Exchange
and ½ Milk Exchange

Ingredients: 2 cups cooked macaroni
4 ozs. grated cheese
salt and pepper to taste
½ tsp. dry mustard
1 tsp. grated onion, if desired
2 cups milk

Method: 1. In bottom of a casserole dish place a layer of cooked macaroni. Cover with half of the cheese, seasonings, and dry mustard, and half of the milk.
2. Repeat layer of macaroni, cheese and seasonings.
3. Add the remainder of the milk.
4. Bake in moderate oven (350°F) until the mixture bubbles and the cheese is melted.

Note: 1. If the meat allowance for the meal is 2 Exchanges (2 ozs.), 8 ozs. cheese could be used in the recipe, and this would make the Exchange per serving:
2 Meat Exchanges
and 1 Bread Exchange
and ½ Milk Exchange
2. If only 4 ozs. cheese are used in the recipe, allow 3 strips crisp bacon or one slice cold meat for the second meat exchange.

WIENERS AND BEANS

Yield: 4 servings

Exchange 1 serving for: 2 Meat Exchanges
and ½ Bread Exchange List 4

Ingredients: 1 cup cooked navy beans
½ cup tomato juice
seasonings to taste
8 wieners

Method: 1. Place beans in casserole. Add heated tomato juice and seasonings.
2. Arrange wieners on top of casserole.
3. Place in moderate oven (350°F) and bake for 15 to 20 minutes, or until wieners are slightly brown and tomato juice is bubbling.

BAKED WIENERS

Yield: 4 servings

Exchange 1 serving for: 2 Meat Exchanges
and 1 Vegetable Exchange List 2A
and 1 Foods as desired

Ingredients: 3 cups canned tomatoes
2 whole cloves
½ clove garlic
1 bay leaf
¼ cup chopped green pepper
¼ cup chopped celery
salt and pepper to taste
8 wieners

Method: 1. Combine tomatoes, garlic, cloves and bay leaf.
2. Simmer uncovered ¾ hour.
3. Add green pepper and celery and simmer an additional 15 minutes.
4. Remove bay leaf and cloves.
5. Place wieners in casserole; pour sauce over top.
6. Bake uncovered, in moderate oven (350°F), for 15 minutes.

Variations: 1. Cut wieners in 1″ pieces and heat in sauce on top of stove.

CHILI CON CARNE

Yield: 4 servings

Exchange 1 serving for: 2 Meat Exchanges
and 1 Bread Exchange
and 1 Vegetable Exchange List 2A

Ingredients: 1½ cups ground lean beaf
2 tbsps. chopped onion
3 cups canned tomatoes
4 drops Tabasco sauce
1 tsp. salt
1 cup cooked red kidney beans

Method: 1. Brown beef over medium heat, preferably in 2 quart "top-of-range" casserole dish, stirring to separate the meat.
2. Add onion, canned tomatoes, Tabasco sauce and salt.
3. Cover and simmer 1 hour, stirring occasionally.
4. Add kidney beans and reheat before serving.

63

SAUSAGE-APPLE ONION BAKE

Yield: 4 servings

Exchange 1 serving for: 3 Meat Exchanges
and 1 Vegetable Exchange List 2B
and 1 Fruit Exchange
and 1 Foods as desired

Ingredients: 4 medium-sized onions
1 tsp. salt
¼ tsp. monosodium glutamate
2¼ cups sausage meat
2 medium, tart apples
1 tsp. salt
½ tsp. nutmeg
½ tsp. artificial liquid sweetener
2 tbsps. orange juice

Method:
1. Cut onions in ¼" slices; cover with boiling water; add salt and monosodium glutamate; boil 5 minutes; drain.
2. Shape sausage meat into patties and pan broil until browned.
3. Wash and core apples and cut into ¼" cross-wise slices; mix with cooked onions, and arrange in bottom of a 2 quart casserole dish.
4. Mix salt, nutmeg, artificial liquid sweetener, and orange juice; drizzle over the apple mixture and arrange browned sausage patties on top.
5. Cover tightlly and bake in moderate oven (350°F) for 25 minutes. Uncover and bake 15 to 20 minutes or until apples are tender.

BEEF CASSEROLE

Yield: 6 servings

Exchange 1 serving for: 3 Meat Exchanges
and 1 Bread Exchange
and 1 Fat Exchange

Ingredients: 1½ lbs. round steak
2 tbsps. fat
6 medium onions
3 cups hot water
1 bay leaf
2½ cups diced carrots
1½ cup raws green beans (cut in strips)
salt and pepper to taste

Method: 1. Wipe meat with a clean damp cloth and cut into 1" pieces.
2. Melt fat in casserole dish over medium heat; add meat, and brown slowly on all sides.
3. During browning of meat, add 2 of the onions which have been thinly sliced. Finish browning the meat.
4. Slowly add hot water and 1 bay leaf. Cover casserole dish and simmer 1½ hours.
5. If necessary, add more water as meat cooks.
6. Add the 4 remaining onions, quartered, and carrots and beans.
7. Cover casserole dish and cook in moderate oven (350°F) ¾ hour or until vegetables are tender.
8. Remove bay leaf before serving.

TUNA FISH AND RICE CASSEROLE

Yield: 4 servings

Exchange 1 serving for: 2 Meat Exchanges
and 1 Bread Exchange

Ingredients: 2 cups canned flaked tuna fish
¾ cup canned condensed cream of mushroom soup, undiluted
¾ cup cooked, drained rice
2 tsps. lemon juice
salt and pepper to taste
water

Method: 1. Mix first 5 ingredients together.
2. Add water to moisten (1/3 to ½ cup).
3. Place mixture in a casserole dish and bake in moderate oven (325°F to 350°F) until it bubbles.
4. Serve hot.

Variations: 1. Salmon or diced cooked chicken may be used in place of the tuna fish.
2. If the fat alowance is sufficient; 1 tsp. of butter per serving may be used to dot the top of the casserole, or if you like ripe olives, 3 medium ripe olives per serving may be sliced into the tuna fish mixture. If you use either butter or the ripe olives, exchange 1 serving for: 2 Meat Exchanges
and 1 Bread Exchange
and 1 Fat Exchange

TUNA FISH AND NOODLE CASSEROLE

Yield: 4 servings

Exchange 1 serving for: 2 Meat Exchanges
and 1 Bread Exchange

Ingredients: 2 cups canned flaked tuna fish
1 and 1/3 cups cooked noodles
1 cup clear chicken broth
seasoning to taste

Method:
1. Combine ingredients.
2. Place in a one quart casserole dish.
3. Bake in moderate oven (350°F) for ½ hour, or until bubbling hot.

Variations:
1. Use flaked salmon, crab, or lobster in place of tuna fish or replace each Meat Exchange with five medium shrimp.
2. Add chopped green pepper or pimento from Vegetable Exchange List 2A.
3. Add a combination of chopped vegetables from Vegetable Exchange List 2A e.g. 2 tbsps. celery, 1 green onion, plus ¼ green pepper.

SALMON CASSEROLE

Yield: 4 servings

Exchange 1 serving for: 2 Meat Exchanges
and ½ Milk Exchange
and 1 Foods as desired

Ingredients: 4 medium sized eggs
2 cups milk
salt and pepper to taste
1 cup flaked, cooked or canned salmon
½ medium onion, grated

Method:
1. Beat egg; add milk, salt and pepper, and mix well.
2. Mix grated onion with the salmon.
3. Add salmon to the milk and egg mixture, and again mix well.
4. Pour into a one-quart casserole dish or into four individual casserole dishes.
5. Place casserole in a pan with 1″ of hot water in the bottom
6. Bake, until set (300° to 325°F), for about ¾ hour.

SALMON AND CELERY CASSEROLE

Yield: 4 servings

Exchange 1 serving for: 1 Meat Exchange
and 1 Vegetable Exchange List 2B

Ingredients: 1 cup canned salmon
¾ cup canned condensed cream of celery soup, undiluted
salt and pepper to taste

Method: 1. Combine ingredients.
2. Place in a casserole dish.
3. Bake in moderate oven (325°F to 350°F) until browned.

Note: ¼ cup to ½ cup water may be used to dilute the soup, if desired, before mixing with the salmon.

GROUND BEEF CASSEROLE

Yield: 4 servings

Exchange 1 serving for: 2 Meat Exchanges
and 1 Vegetable Exchange List 2A

Ingredients: 1½ cups (or 1 lb.) raw ground beef
1 and 1/3 cups canned tomatoes
¼ cup green pepper, chopped or sliced
1 tbsp. chopped onion
salt and pepper to taste

Method: 1. Brown ground beef over high heat, stirring to separate it.
2. Place half the meat in bottom of a one-quart casserole dish.
3. Then place half the onion and green pepper on top.
4. Season.
5. Add half the tomatoes.
6. Add the remainder of the minced beef, onions, and green pepper, and pour the remaining tomatoes over the mixture.
7. Bake ½ to ¾ hour at 350°F.

Suggestions for serving:

1. Use 1/3 cup cooked rice, spaghetti, or noodles as 1 Bread Exchange.
2. Use leftover minced beef or ham in place of the raw beef.
3. In summer, fresh tomatoes may be used, sliced in layers between the meat, in place of canned tomatoes. Use four medium-sized tomatoes in place of 1 and 1/3 cups canned tomatoes.

67

CHICKEN AND RICE CASSEROLE

Yield: 4 servings

Exchange 1 serving for: 2 Meat Exchanges
and 1 Bread Exchange

Ingredients: 2 cups cooked diced chicken
1 and 1/3 cups cooked rice
1 cup clear chicken broth
salt and pepper to taste

Method: 1. Combine the ingredients.
2. Place in a one-quart casserole dish or divide evenly into four individual casserole dishes, if desired.
3. Bake in a moderate oven (350°F) until bubbling hot.

Variations: 1. Add chopped parsley or mushrooms. They may be used freely.
2. Add chopped celery, green pepper, pimento, or onion from Vegetable Exchange List 2A.

CHICKEN NOODLE CASSEROLE

Yield: 4 servings

Exchange 1 serving for: 1 Bread Exchange
and 2 Meat Exchanges
and 1 Fat Exchange

Ingredients: 1 and 1/3 cups cooked noodles
2 cups diced cooked chicken
1 cup clear chicken broth
4 tsps. butter or margarine
salt and pepper to taste

Method: 1. Combine the ingredients in a casserole dish.
2. Brown in moderate oven (325°F to 350°F).

Variations: 1. Use equal amounts of rice or spaghetti in place of noodles.
2. Mushrooms (may be used freely) and green pepper (Vegetable Exchange List 2A) may be added.
3. Any cooked meat or fish may be used to replace the chicken.

CHICKEN A LA KING

Yield: 4 servings

Exchange 1 serving (without toast) for: 3 Meat Exchanges
and 1 Bread Exchange

Ingredients: 8 mushrooms, sliced
½ cup clear chicken broth
2 cups skim milk or reconstituted nonfat dry milk
¼ cup flour
½ tsp. salt
dash of pepper
1 tbsp. chopped pimento
3 cups diced cooked chicken

Method:
1. Cook mushroms in broth.
2. Drain and measure broth; add water to make ½ cup.
3. Heat 1½ cups milk and ½ cup broth in top of a double boiler.
4. Blend flour and the remaining ½ cup skim milk until no lumps remain.
5. Add to heated milk and broth, stirring constantly until thickened, over the boiling water.
6. Add chicken, mushrooms, pimento and seasonings.
7. Reheat.
8. Serve in individual casserole dishes or on toast. (Add necessary Bread Exchange if toast is used.)

Variations:
1. Use ½ cup skim milk powder and 2¼ cups chicken broth as liquid.
2. If whole milk is used, the exchange per serving is **increased by** 1 Fat Exchange.

BEEF AND SPAGHETTI CASSEROLE

Yield: 4 servings

Exchange 1 serving for: 2 Meat Exchanges
and 1 Bread Exchange
and 1 Vegetable Exchange List 2 A

Ingredients: 2 cups minced or diced cooked beef
1 and 1/3 cups cooked spaghetti
1 and 1/3 cups tomato juice
salt and pepper to taste

Method: 1. Combine the ingredients.
2. Place in a one-quart or four individual casserole dishes.
3. Bake in oven at 350°F for 1/2 hour.

Variations: 1. Use canned or fresh tomatoes in place of tomato juice.
2. Add a dash of Tabasco sauce to tomato juice in place of pepper.
3. Add celery or green pepper from Vegetable Exchange List 2A.
4. Replace 1/4 cup minced or diced beef with 1/4 cup grated cheese. Sprinkle cheese over casserole before baking.

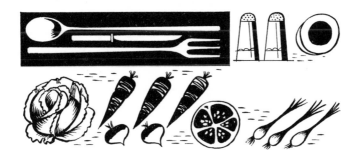

SALADS

Salads are often the bright spots in our meals. With their crisp green and colorful vegetables and fruits, they can tempt the dullest appetite. For diabetics, they are especially important, since they provide essential roughage, minerals, and vitamins in addition to the necessary measured amounts of their nutrients. Some salads serve as appetizers or main course accompaniments. Others are heartier and may take the place of the main dish at luncheon or supper. Whatever their role in the menu plan, salads should be fresh, simple, colorful and attractive and should taste good! The salad planned for the diabetic can represent a vegetable exchange, a fruit exchange, a meat exchange, a fat exchange, or any combination of these, plus many of the free foods. Salad-making is an artistic challenge, and it can be a pleasure when a few rules are carefully followed.

How To Choose Your Salad Ingredients:

Many small salads and salad garnishes may be chosen from the Vegetable Exchange List 2A The familiar tossed salad, combining several raw vegetables and a suitable dressing, is always in good taste, and gives scope for plenty of variety. Vegetables from Vegetable Exchange List 2B can be used raw or cooked, to make additional varieties of mixed salads.

When using a Vegetable Exchange for a salad, you will get more variety by considering the exchange in two, three, or four parts. By referring to your Exchange lists, you can estimate $\frac{1}{4}$ of the amounts for four different vegetables, and these can be combined to make a delicious salad.

Example: ¼ raw tomato (medium size)

¼ green pepper (medium size)

⅛ cup shredded raw cabbage

1 large leaf lettuce

will equal 1 Vegetable Exchange List 2A The tomato and pepper can be chopped and combined with the cabbage, a dressing added if desired (and if allowed), and this can be served on the crisp lettuce leaf.

Additional suggested combinations from Vegetable Exchange List 2A include:

— lettuce, cucumber, celery, and green pepper.

— chicory, tomato, and radish.

— lettuce, parsley, raw cauliflower, and tomato.

— endive, tomato, and cucumber.

— cabbage, celery, and green pepper.

— lettuce, watercress, and cucumber.

— lettuce, raw spinach, and radish.

Similarly, a Fruit Exchange can be divided to include two or more fruits. But, any part of the Fruit Exchange should **not** be substituted for a part of a Vegetable Exchange and vice versa. Each type of exchange must be calculated separately, even though the foods are finally combined into a mixed salad.

When meat, fish, poultry, cheese or eggs are used in a main course salad, these must also be calculated in terms of a Meat Exchange. In making jellied salads, plain gelatin or artificially sweetened jelly powders should be used, so that exchange values are not affected.

Since most salads are marinated or garnished with a dressing, it is important to remember to calculate the value of the dressing. A simple oil and vinegar dressing, a French dressing, or a mayonnaise dressing may be used, depending upon the amount needed and the fat allowance in your meal plan.

General Rules For Salad Preparation

1. All ingredients, including greens, fruits and vegetables, should be fresh and of good quality.
2. Use fruits and vegetables in season whenever possible, for best quality, flavor and economy.
3. Wash and trim lettuce and celery as soon as you return from shopping. Store in plastic bags or covered containers in the refrigerator.
4. Wash, trim and drain watercress, parsley, radishes, etc. and store in crisper or covered containers in refrigerator.
5. Wash and trim cabbage, crisp in ice water and drain before using.
6. To retain crispness, greens and other fresh vegetables and fruits should be mixed with dressing just before serving. Cooked vegetables, meats, fish and poultry may be marinated ahead of serving time to improve flavor of the salad mixture.
7. Retain the fresh, natural color of peeled or sliced fruits (pears, peaches and apples) by covering them with water to which salt, lemon juice or vinegar has been added. Drain well before using.

Salad Garnishes

The garnish on the salad should be simple, but should complement the ingredients by making them more attractive and palatable. There is an old-fashioned rule which says, "Every garnish must be edible." You'll agree this seems a sensible guide in all food preparation. The Foods used freely should be chosen as garnishes whenever possible. In addition, small portions of vegetables from Vegetable Exchange List 2A may be allowed for garnishes. The following suggestions will help you to choose:

Foods—Little Calorie Value:

Horseradish; lemon; parsley; mint; cranberries.

Foods to be used freely in quantities shown.

Catsup (1 tsp.); lemon juice (1 tbsp.); prepared mustard (1 tsp.); lemon wedge or twists; dill pickle (1 med.); sour pickles (4 pieces); dietetic sweet mixed pickles (4 pieces); pimento or chopped green pepper (1 tbsp.).

Vegetable Exchange — List 2A or 2B

Small portions of the following: Celery heart, stick or fan; green pepper diamonds, strip or rings; cucumber sticks, twists or fluted slices; 1 small green onion; 1 slice onion, or 1 tsp. chopped onion; radish roses, slices or fans; thin slice or small wedge of tomato; small serving of lettuce.

Salad Dressings

Study your Fat Exchange List.

If your meal plan includes enough Fat Exchanges to allow a dressing on your salad, keep the following points in mind:
1. One tsp. of vegetable oil provides 1 Fat Exchange, and it may be mixed with vinegar or lemon juice and herbs, or seasonings to make a tasty dressing.
2. One tbsp. of commercial French dressing provides 1 Fat Exchange.
3. One tsp. of commercial mayonnaise provides 1 Fat Exchange.
4. One rounded tbsp. of whipped cream, with artificial liquid sweetener, provides 1 Fat Exchange, as used on a fruit salad.
5. One tbsp. lemon juice may be used to dress greens or tossed salad mixtures.

FRUIT SALAD DRESSING

Yield: ½ cup

Exchange 1 tbsp. for: 1 Foods used freely

Ingredients: 1 tbsp. gelatin
1 tbsp. cold water
¼ cup boiling water
1 tbsp. artificial liquid sweetener
¼ tsp. salt
¼ cup lemon juice
⅛ tsp. dry mustard
½ tsp. paprika

Method: 1. Soften gelatin in cold water; dissolve in boiling water.
2. Combine remaining ingredients and mix with dissolved gelatin. Store in refrigerator. Becomes firm when cold. Reheat to liquify.

LEMON JUICE DRESSING

Yield: 1⅛ cups

Exchange 1 tbsp. for: 1 Foods used freely

Ingredients: ½ cup lemon juice
2 tbsps. salad oil
½ cup water
½ tsp. salt
¼ tsp. pepper
½ tsp. celery salt
¼ tsp. dry mustard

Method:
1. Beat the lemon juice into the salad oil.
2. Add gradually ½ cup water.
3. Add the salt, pepper, celery salt and mustard. Chill.
4. Beat or shake vigorously before using.

TOMATO FRENCH DRESSING

Yield: 1 cup

Exchange 1 tbsp. for: ½ Vegetable Exchange List 2A

Ingredients: ½ cup canned condensed tomato soup, undiluted
¼ cup water
2 tbsps. vinegar
1 tbsp. grated onion
2 tbsps. finely chopped green pepper
1 tsp. Worcestershire sauce
½ tsp. salt
½ tsp. dry mustard
⅛ tsp. garlic powder
¼ tsp. artificial liquid sweetener

Method:
1. Beat all ingredients together until smooth, preferably in an electric blender.
2. Shake well before using.

BOILED DRESSING

Yield: 1 cup

Exchange 1 tbsp. for: 1 Foods used freely

Ingredients: 2/3 cup skim milk or reconstituted nonfat dry milk
2 eggs
1 tsp. salt
½ tsp. paprika
½ tsp. dry mustard
dash of cayenne pepper
2 tbsps. cider vinegar

Method:
1. Beat eggs lightly in top of a double boiler.
2. Blend in milk, salt, spices and vinegar.
3. Place over hot water.
4. Cook, stirring constantly until thickened.
5. Chill before serving.

MAYONNAISE

Yield: 1 cup

Exchange 1 tbsp. for: ½ Fat Exchange

Ingredients: 2 eggs
¾ tsp. salt
½ tsp. paprika
¼ tsp. dry mustard
3 tbsps. lemon juice
½ cup milk
1 tbsp. salad oil

Method:
1. Beat eggs, salt, paprika and mustard in the top of a double boiler.

2. Gradually add the milk and lemon juice.

3. Place over hot water. Cook, stirring constantly until thickened.

4. Remove from the heat and stir in the salad oil.

5. Chill, and keep refrigerated.

WALDORF SALAD

Yield: 1 serving

Exchange for: 1 Fruit Exchange
and 1 Fat Exchange
and ½ Vegetable Exchange List 2A

Ingredients: ½ medium-sized apple, brightly colored
¼ cup diced raw celery
1 tsp. mayonnaise, diluted with a little lemon juice

Method:
1. Leaving skin on, wash apple and cut in half.

2. Remove core, stem and calyx, and cut ½ apple into small cubes.

3. Add diced celery and mayonnaise, diluted with lemon juice.

4. Mix thoroughly and marinate for a few minutes before serving.

5. Serve on a crisp lettuce cup.

POTATO SALAD

Yield: 1 serving

Exchange for: 1 Bread Exchange
or 2 Vegetable Exchanges List 2 B

Ingredients: 1 small chilled, boiled potato
½ tsp. finely chopped onion
1 tsp. chopped pimento
dressing to moisten (see recipes and exchange values)
salt and pepper to taste

Method: 1. Dice potato and mix with other ingredients.
2. Chill well before using.

Note: Check values of dressing used and add 1 Fat Exchange, if necessary, to account for dressing used.

Variations: 1. Small amounts of chopped celery, parsley or green pepper may be added without altering exchange values.
2. Add 1 hard-cooked egg, sliced, or ¼ cup diced ham or bologna, or 5 small shrimps, and increase Exchange value by adding 1 Meat Exchange.

DEVILED EGGS

Yield: 1 egg (2 halves) equals 1 serving

Exchange 1 egg for: 1 Meat Exchange
Add 1 Fat Exchange if commercial mayonnaise is used

Ingredients: 1 hard-cooked egg
salt and other seasonings
pinch of dry mustard
salad dressing to moisten
paprika for garnish

Method: 1. Peel and cut egg either crosswise or lengthwise.
2. Remove yolk and mash with a fork.
3. Add salt, seasonings and mustard to egg yolk.
4. Moisten with salad dressing.
5. Refill egg white with yolk mixture.
6. Garnish with paprika.

CHICKEN, SALMON, OR TUNA FISH SALAD

Yield: 1 serving

Exchange for: 2 Meat Exchanges
Add 1 Fat Exchange if commercial dressing is used

Ingredients: ½ cup diced, cooked chicken, or drained flaked salmon or tuna fish
1 tbsp. chopped celery
1 tsp. chopped onion or green pepper, if desired
salt and pepper to taste
salad dressing to moisten

Method: 1. Combine all ingredients.
2. Chill and serve with green salad or lettuce.

GELATIN SALADS

Using unflavored gelatin or artificially sweetened jelly powders as bases, a variety of delicious jellied salads may be made. Exchange values of the salads will depend upon the ingredients. Jellied salads should be well chilled and kept cold until serving time.

BASIC JELLY FOR SALADS

Yield: 6 servings

Exchange 1 serving for: 1 Foods used freely, if plain
Add Exchange value of all added ingredients, such as vegetables, fruit, meat, fish or poultry.

Ingredients: 1 envelope unflavored gelatin
1¾ cups water
¼ tsp. salt
½ tsp. mixed spices
¼ cup diluted vinegar or lemon juice

Method: 1. Sprinkle gelatin into ½ cup cold water to soften.
2. Bring remaining water to boil, and add the other ingredients.
3. Strain to remove spices.
4. Add softened gelatin and stir until thoroughly dissolved.
5. Chill to consistency of unbeaten egg white, before adding measured amounts of vegetables, fruit, meat or fish.
6. Chill until firm. Unmold just befor serving.

Note: Artificial liquid sweetener may be added to taste, if desired.

TOMATO ASPIC

Yield: 6 servings (½ cup each)

Exchange 1 serving for: ½ Vegetable Exchange List 2A

Ingredients: 1 envelope unflavored gelatin
½ cup cold water
2 cups cooked or canned tomatoes
¼ bay leaf
1 clove
1 tbsp. vinegar or lemon juice
½ tbsp. chopped celery
10 chopped olives

Method: 1. Sprinkle gelatin into cold water to soften.
2. Bring tomatoes and spices to a boil.
3. Dissolve softened gelatin in the hot mixture.
4. Add vinegar or lemon juice.
5. Strain and discard spices and seeds.
6. Chill until partially set.
7. Stir in chopped vegetables and olives.
8. Pour into one large mold or 6 individual molds.
9. Chill until firm.

Note: Artificial liquid sweetener may be added to taste if desired.

TOMATO ASPIC MADE WITH TOMATO JUICE

Yield: 2 servings

Exchange 1 serving for: 1 Vegetable Exchange List 2A

Ingredients: 1 cup tomato juice
dash of salt
dash of celery salt
1 tsp. chopped onion
1 whole clove
small piece of bay leaf
2 tsps. vinegar
1 envelope artificially sweetened lemon jelly powder

Method: 1. Combine tomato juice and all seasonings in a saucepan.
2. Cover and bring to a boil.
3. Remove from heat and pour over artificially sweetened jelly powder, stirring until dissolved.
4. Cover and let stand 5 minutes.
5. Strain and divide evenly into 2 molds.
6. Chill until firm.

GRAPEFRUIT CRESS SALAD

Yield: 2 servings

Exchange 1 serving for: ½ Fruit Exchange

Ingredients: 1 envelope artificially sweetened lemon jelly powder
dash of salt
1 cup hot water
5 sections drained, unsweetened grapefruit sections
¼ cup coarsely cut watercress or celery tops
½ tsp. drained chopped pimento

Method:
1. Dissolve jelly powder and salt in hot water.
2. Chill until slightly thickened.
3. Fold in grapefruit sections, cut in half, watercress and pimento.
4. Divide evenly into 2 molds.
5. Chill until firm.
6. Unmold on crisp salad greens.
7. Serve with dressing, if allowed.

CONFETTI SALAD

Yield: 2 servings

Exchange 1 serving for: ½ Vegetable Exchange List 2A

Ingredients: 1 envelope artificially sweetened lemon jelly powder
1 cup hot water
⅛ tsp. salt
¼ tsp. grated onion
¼ cup very small pieces of raw cauliflower or shredded cabbage
2 tsps. diced pimento

Method:
1. Dissolve jelly powder in hot water.
2. Add salt and onion.
3. Chill until slightly thickened.
4. Fold in cauliflower and pimento.
5. Divide evenly into 2 molds.
6. Chill until firm.
7. Unmold on crisp greens.
8. Serve with low-calorie mayonnaise or dressing.

APPLE CIDER SALAD

Yield: 6 servings

Exchange 1 serving for: 2 Fruit Exchanges

Ingredients: 1½ tbsps, unflavored gelatin
1/3 cup cold water
2 tsps. artificial liquid sweetener
2 cups apple cider or apple juice
2 tbsps. lemon juice
½ tsp. salt
2 medium-sized apples, finely chopped

Method: 1. Soften gelatin in cold water.
2. Combine artificial liquid sweetener, cider, lemon juice and salt.
3. Heat and add to the softened gelatin, stirring until gelatin is dissolved.
4. Cool until mixture begins to thicken.
5. Fold in apples.
6. Pour into a 3-cup mold or divide into 6 individual molds.
7. Chill until firm.
8. Unmold on crisp greens.

JELLIED SPRING VEGETABLE SALAD

Yield: 6 servings

Exchange 1 serving for: ½ Vegetable Exchange List 2A

Ingredients: 1 tbsp. unflavored gelatin
¼ cup cold water
2 cups boiling water
½ tsp. salt
¼ cup unsweetened lime juice
2 tsps. artificial liquid sweetener
few drops green food coloring
1 cup diced, peeled cucumber
1 cup sliced radishes
¼ cup sliced green onions

Method: 1. Soften gelatin in cold water; dissolve in boiling water.
2. Add salt, lime juice, and artificial liquid sweetener.
3. Chill until mixture begins to thicken.
4. Fold in remaining ingredients.
5. Pour into a 3-cup mold or divide into 6 individual molds.
6. Chill until firm, and unmold on crisp greens.

GRAPE AND GRAPEFRUIT GELATIN SALAD

Yield: 2 servings

Exchange 1 serving for: ½ Fruit Exchange

Ingredients: 1 tsp. unflavored gelatin
2 tbsps. cold water
5 tbsps. hot water
2 tbsps. grape juice (unsweetened)
¼ grapefruit, cut into sections
1 tsp. lemon juice
one ¼-grain tablet artificial sweetener

Method: 1. Soften gelatin in cold water.
2. Heat grape juice with hot water; add to gelatin, and stir until dissolved.
3. Cool.
4. Dissolve sweetener in lemon juice and add to gelatin mixture.
5. Pour into a mold, and when mixture begins to set add the grapefruit sections.
6. Chill until firm, and unmold on crisp greens.

JELLIED CHICKEN AND VEGETABLE SALAD

Yield: 4 servings

Exchange 1 serving for: 1 Meat Exchange
and 1 Vegetable Exchange List 2 A

Ingredients: 1 envelope unflavored gelatin
¼ cup cold water
2 cups fat-free chicken stock
1 cup (4 ozs.) cooked, diced chicken
2 cups of diced celery, green pepper, sliced radishes, and asparagus tips combined

Method: 1. Soften gelatin in cold water.
2. Add hot chicken stock and stir until dissolved.
3. Pour a thin layer of liquid jelly into a mold. Let this set slightly.
4. Add a layer of vegetables, then a layer of diced chicken.
5. Add another thin layer of liquid jelly and let it set slightly.
6. Continue these layers until all vegetables, chicken and jelly mixture are used.
7. Chill until firm. Unmold and place on a lettuce leaf.

LIME COTTAGE CHEESE SALAD

Yield: 4 servings
Exchange 1 serving for: ½ Meat Exchange
Ingredients: 2 envelopes artificially sweetened lime jelly powder
2 cups hot water
2 tsps. vinegar
⅛ tsp. salt
½ cup cottage cheese
2 tsps. pimento
1 tsp. grated onion
Method: 1. Dissolve jelly powder in hot water.
2. Stir in vinegar and salt
3. Pour 1 cup of this mixture into a mold.
4. Chill until almost firm.
5. At the same time, chill remaining cup of jelly base until slightly thickened.
6. Into it, fold cheese, pimento and onion.
7. Pour over first jelly layer in mold.
8. Chill until firm, and unmold on crisp greens.

PERFECTION SALAD

Yield: 4 servings
Exchange 1 serving for: ½ Vegetable Exchange List 2A
Ingredients: 1/3 cup diluted vinegar
1 and 1/3 cups boiling water
¾ tsp. salt
½ tsp. artificial liquid sweetener
1 and 1/3 tbsps. unflavored gelatin
1/3 cup cold water
juice of 1 lemon
2/3 cup shredded cabbage
1½ cups diced celery
2 tbsps. chopped green pepper or pimento
1 or 2 drops green food coloring, if desired
Method: 1. Mix boiling water, vinegar, and salt; heat to boiling point.
2. Soften gelatin in cold water; dissolve in boiling liquid after it is removed from the stove.
3. Add lemon juice and artificial liquid sweetener.
4. When slightly thickened, add vegetables.
5. Divide into four moistened molds. Chill until firm.

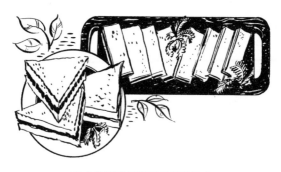

SANDWICHES

Ever since the Earl of Sandwich first introduced his novel idea, its popularity has grown. Many people carry sandwiches in lunch boxes to school, to work, or on picnics. At afternoon teas or evening parties, sandwiches, hot or cold, plain or fancy, large or small, are often more attractive than the cakes. This trend should please the diabetic, who will have to forego the cake, but can pick and choose from the sandwich tray.

Included on the following pages are suggestions for sandwich fillings which may be made at home, but which can also be ordered from a restaurant menu. In addition, suggestions are included for hamburgers and hot dogs.

The amount of bread or roll used in making the sandwiches, hamburgers or hot dogs will depend on the bread allowance for the meal. Many of the fillings make up well in an open-faced sandwich which requires only one slice of bread or ½ hamburger bun or ½ wiener roll.

EGG SALAD SANDWICH FILLING

Yield: 1 serving

Exchange for: 1 Meat Exchange
and 1 Fat Exchange

Ingredients: 1 egg, hard cooked
pinch of dry mustard
½ tsp. chopped onion, celery, or green pepper
1 tsp. mayonnaise
salt and pepper to taste

Method: 1. Mash egg with a fork.
2. Add seasonings, mayonnaise, chopped onion, etc.
3. Mix well. Refrigerate until time of using.

SALMON, TUNA OR LOBSTER FILLING

Yield: 1 serving

Exchange for: 1 Meat Exchange
and 1 Fat Exchange

Ingredients: ¼ cup of cooked or canned salmon, tuna, or lobster
1 tsp. chopped celery
½ tsp. chopped onion for flavoring if desired
1 tsp. mayonnaise
lemon juice or vinegar
salt and pepper to taste

Method: 1. Flake the fish with a fork.
2. Mix well with the other ingredients.
3. Refrigerate until time of using.

Note: The mayonnaise may be omitted if desired, in which case the exchange for the filling would be only 1 Meat Exchange.

CHICKEN SALAD SANDWICH FILLING

Yield: 1 serving

Exchange for: 1 Meat Exchange
and 1 Fat Exchange

Ingredients: ¼ cup cooked chopped, or minced chicken
1 tsp. chopped celery
1 tsp. mayonnaise
salt and pepper to taste

Method: 1. Mix all ingredients until well blended.
2. Refrigerate until time of using.

MINCED BEEF, VEAL, OR HAM FILLING

Yield: 1 serving

Exchange for: 1 Meat Exchange
and 1 Fat Exchange

Ingredients: ¼ cup minced beef, veal, or ham
½ tsp. chopped onion
½ tsp. chopped unsweetened pickle
pinch of mustard, if desired
1 tsp. mayonnaise
salt and pepper to taste

Method: 1. Mix all ingredients until well blended.
2. Refrigerate until time of using.

85

COLD SLICED CHICKEN, BEEF, VEAL, LAMB, OR HAM FILLING

Yield: 1 serving
Exchange for: 2 Meat Exchanges
Ingredients: 2 slices of any of the above meats, each slice measuring
       4″ x 2″ x ¼″
       salt and pepper to taste
       lettuce, if desired
Note: With beef, a little horseradish may be used.

With ham or beef, a little mustard may be used — prepared mustard, or home-made mustard.
With chicken, mayonnaise may be used. If mayonnaise is used, the exchange would be: 2 Meat Exchanges
       and 1 Fat Exchange

GRILLED CHEESE SANDWICH

Yield: 1 sandwich
Exchange for: 1 Meat Exchange
       and 2 Bread Exchanges
Ingredients: 2 slices bread
       1 slice of pre-sliced processed cheese
Method: 1. Place cheese between two slices of bread.
       2. Toast in sandwich toaster, grill, or brown in hot oven (400°F-425°F), turning during the cooking to brown the bread.

GRILLED CHEESE AND BACON SANDWICH

Yield: 1 sandwich
Exchange for: 2 Meat Exchanges
       and 1 Bread Exchange
Ingredients: 1 slice of pre-sliced processed cheese
       3 strips bacon, partially cooked and cut in half
       1 slice bread
Method: 1. Place cheese on top of bread.
       2. Place partially cooked bacon on top of cheese.
       3. Broil, or finish cooking in hot oven (400°F-425°F) until bacon is cooked and cheese melting.
Note: Ham, or other meat may be used in place of bacon. When meat is used in place of the bacon, place meat next to the bread, and the cheese on top of the meat, with a little catsup or mustard, or slice of tomato on top for extra flavor.

HOT DOG DELIGHT

Yield: 1 serving

Exchange for: 2 Meat Exchanges
and 1 Fat Exchange
and 2 Bread Exchanges

Ingredients: 1 wiener, cooked
1 slice pre-sliced processed cheese
1 strip partially cooked bacon
1 wiener roll

Method:
1. Roll cheese around wiener which has been cooked, and roll the partially cooked bacon around both cheese and wiener.
2. Fasten with a tooth pick.
3. Broil for 1 to 2 minutes.
4. Place on a heated wiener bun.

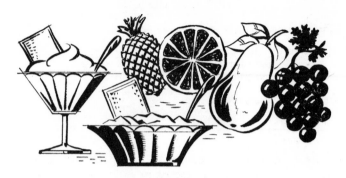

DESSERTS

"The mission of dessert is being that of a comforter of the stomach which being already appeased, nevertheless requires a little reflex flattery."

Desserts have many functions. There is the satisfaction that most people feel in having an attractive sweet at the end of a meal. They also supply nutrients required by a diet. For those who are on dietary restrictions, such as diabetics, there must be careful planning and use. Sweets, as such, do contain high percentages of sugar, so substitutions may have to be made.

Desserts fall into several categories. Fruit is abundantly available. Fresh fruit is often preferred and it can be used any time according to dietary allowances. Other desserts suitable for diabetics include gelatin whips in which fruits are used, and simple milk puddings which may be garnished with some fruit.

Many of these dessert recipes are also suitable for members of the family who are not diabetic.

DESSERTS, Classified According to Exchanges:

A — Milk Exchanges

1. Cocoa Floating Island
2. Apple Mousse
3. Soft Custard
4. Blanc Mange (Cream Pudding)
5. Junket
6. Baked Custard
7. Tapioca Pudding
8. Rice Pudding

B — Fruit Exchanges

1. Pumpkin Custard
2. Apple Snow
3. Apricot Whip
4. Banana Sponge
5. Jellied Fruits
6. Lime Fluff
7. Baked Apple
8. Chocolate Pudding

C — Combined Exchanges

1. Orange Pudding
2. Floating Island
3. Rice Pineapple Dessert
4. Graham Wafer Lemon Tart
5. Plum Pudding Recipe I
6. Plum Pudding Recipe II
7. Tarts
8. Shortcake
9. Dutch Apple Cake
10. Ice Cream Jelly Bavarian

D — Low Calorie

1. Orange Whip
2. Mocha Fluff
3. Coffee Jelly

Sauces

1. Chocolate Sauce
2. Lemon Sauce
3. Orange Sauce

A — Milk Exchanges

When using desserts which are calculated as a Milk Exchange, the fruit allowance for the meal may be used as fruit juice. If milk other than whole milk is used, make exchange for fat as suggested in the pages of general information.

COCOA FLOATING ISLAND

Yield: 6 servings

Exchange 1 serving for: 1/4 Milk Exchange

Ingredients: 2 cups skim milk or reconstituted nonfat dry milk
3 eggs, separated
1/8 tsp. salt
1/2 tsp. vanilla
1 tsp. artificial liquid sweetener
2 tbsps. cocoa

Method:
1. Scald milk.
2. Put egg yolks in the top of a double boiler and beat lightly with a fork; add salt.
3. While stirring, gradually add the hot milk. Place over hot water.
4. Cook, stirring constantly, until the mixture thickens and forms a coating on a silver spoon.
5. Add vanilla and one half of the artificial liquid sweetener.
6. Strain and cool.
7. When ready to serve, beat egg whites until stiff.
8. Add cocoa and other half artificial liquid sweetener.
9. Place a heaping spoonful of this meringue on top of each serving of pudding.

APPLE MOUSSE

Yield: 6 servings

Exchange 1 serving for: ¼ Milk Exchange
and ½ Fruit Exchange

Ingredients: ¾ cup evaporated milk, thoroughly chilled
1½ cups unsweetened apple sauce
1½ tsps. lemon juice
⅜ tsp. salt
⅜ tsp. nutmeg
1½ tsps. artificial liquid sweetener

Method:
1. Whip evaporated milk until stiff. (Do not overwhip)
2. Fold in remaining ingredients.
3. Pour into individual molds, or into a tray, and freeze until firm.
4. Unmold, or cut if in a tray, and serve.

BLANC MANGE (CREAM PUDDING)

Yield: 6 servings

Exchange 1 serving for: ½ Milk Exchange
and 1 Fat Exchange

Ingredients: 2 tbsps. unflavored gelatin
6 tbsps. cold water
2¼ cups milk
¾ cup cream (18%)
6 cloves, whole
⅛ tsp. salt
¾ tsp. cinnamon
¾ tsp. vanilla
1½ tsps. artificial liquid sweetener

Method:
1. Add gelatin to cold water.
2. Boil cloves and cinnamon in ¼ cup hot water for 1 minute.
3. Strain into soaked gelatin — if this is not sufficient to dissolve the gelatin, heat in double boiler over hot water until dissolved.
4. Add milk and cream to dissolved gelatin.
5. Add vanilla, salt and artificial liquid sweetener.
6. Pour into six serving dishes; chill.

Note: May be unmolded and served with either fresh or canned fruit or a fruit sauce, which must be counted as a Fruit Exchange.

WESTERN SANDWICH

Yield: 1 sandwich

Exchange for: 2 Meat Exchanges
and 1 Fat Exchange
and 2 Bread Exchanges

Ingredients: 3 strips crisp bacon, cut into small pieces
or ¼ cup diced cooked ham
1 tsp. chopped onion
1 egg
salt and pepper to taste
2 slices bread or toast

Method: 1. Cook bacon pieces; remove from pan.
2. Drain fat from pan, leaving 1 tsp. in which to cook the chopped onion until lightly browned.
3. Break egg into frying pan; add the cooked bacon pieces, salt and pepper. Stir briskly to mix all ingredients and to keep egg from sticking to the pan. Cook until egg is firm, but not hard.
4. Serve between 2 slices bread or toast.

TOASTED SARDINE SANDWICH

Yield: 1 sandwich

Exchange for: 3 Meat Exchanges
and 1 Bread Exchange
and 1 Fat Exchange

Ingredients: 6 sardines in mustard sauce
1 tsp. butter or margarine
1 slice bread
1 slice pre-sliced processed cheese

Method: 1. Drain sardines. Mix ½ tsp. mustard sauce with softened butter or margarine and spread on bread.
2. Arrange sardines on bread and top with sliced cheese.
3. Sprinkle with paprika.
4. Toast in hot oven (450°F to 500°F) for 8 to 10 minutes, or until cheese begins to melt.

HAM ROLL

Yield: 1 serving

Exchange for: 1 Bread Exchange
and 1 Meat Exchange
and 1 Fat Exchange

Ingredients: ¼ cup minced cooked ham
1 tsp. chopped celery
1 tsp. mayonnaise
salt and pepper to taste
1 parkerhouse roll

Method: 1. Mix first 4 ingredients.
2. Place filling in parkerhouse roll which has been split lengthwise.
3. Place in moderate oven (375°F) about 5 minutes, or until the roll and filling have been heated through.
4. Serve hot.

Note: Chicken or fish filling may be used in place of the ham and in the same amount.

HAMBURGER

Yield: 1 serving

Exchange for: 2 Meat Exchanges
and 2 Bread Exchanges
and 1 Fat Exchange

Ingredients: 6 tbsps. raw lean ground beef
salt and pepper to taste
1 tsp. butter or margarine
1 hamburger bun

Method: 1. Form seasoned minced beef into a meat patty.
2. Broil in oven or pan broil on top of stove.
3. Split and butter bun and warm in oven if desired.
4. Place meat patty in bun and serve hot with one or more of the following, according to Dietary allowance:

1. 1 slice tomato — 1 Vegetable Exchange List 2A.
2. 1 slice onion — ½ Vegetable Exchange List 2B.
3. Cole slaw, 1/3 to ½ cup — 1 Vegetable Exchange List 2B
4. 1 tsp. catsup — 1 Foods as desired
5. ½ to 1 tsp. mustard — 1 Foods used freely
6. 3 or 4 slices unsweetened dill pickles — 1 Foods as desired

Variations: The meat patty may be varied without appreciably changing its exchange value by adding to the minced beef before broiling one or two of the following:

½ tsp. finely chopped onion
½ tsp. finely chopped green pepper
¼ tsp. Worcestershire sauce
⅛ to ¼ tsp. horseradish
½ tsp. hamburger relish

CHEESEBURGER

Yield: 1 serving
Exchange for: 2 Meat Exchanges
and 1 Bread Exchange
and 2 Fat Exchanges
Ingredients: 3 tbsps. raw lean ground beef
½ tsp. grated onion, if desired
salt and pepper to taste
1 tsp. butter or margarine
1 slice pre-sliced processed cheese
1 strip side bacon
½ hamburger bun
Method: 1. Add grated onion and seasonings to the raw lean ground beef and shape into a meat patty.
2. Cook under broiler, or if desired, cook in frying pan with the 1 tsp. butter or margarine and a little water, if necessary, to keep it from sticking to the pan.
3. Place the cooked meat patty on half hamburger bun.
4. Top with slice of cheese and then the strip of bacon, cut in half.
5. Place in oven under broiler until the bacon is cooked. If you do not have a broiler, partially cook the bacon before placing it on top of the cheese, and then put the cheeseburger in a hot oven (400°F to 425°F) until the bacon is cooked.

Note: 1 tsp. butter or margarine has been allowed. It may be used when (1) cooking the meat patty or (2) to butter the bun or (3) it may be omitted entirely. If it is omitted, the exchange of fat would only be ONE instead of two Fat Exchanges. If the meal plan allows 2 Bread Exchanges, a whole hamburger bun may be used instead of ½ bun. The top of the bun should not be put on the cheeseburger until the bacon is cooked.

TUNA BURGERS

Yield: 6 servings

Exchange 1 serving for: 2 Meat Exchanges
and 2 Bread Exchanges
and 2 Fat Exchanges
and 1 Vegetable Exchange List 2A

Ingredients: one 7-oz. can tuna fish, drained and flaked
¾ cup chopped celery
1 small onion, diced
½ cup diced cheese
½ cup chopped olives
3 tbsps. mayonnaise
salt and pepper to taste
6 hamburger buns

Method:
1. Mix tuna fish, celery, onion, cheese, olives, mayonnaise, salt and pepper.
2. Split 6 hamburger buns.
3. Divide the tuna filling evenly among the six buns.
4. Place the buns in dampened paper sandwich bags or wrap in aluminum foil folding and fastening with paper clips.
5. Heat in moderate oven (350°F) 15 to 20 minutes.
6. Serve hot.

HOT DOG

Yield: 1 serving

Exchange for: 1 Meat Exchange
and 2 Bread Exchanges

Ingredients: 1 wiener
1 wiener roll
½ to 1 tsp. mustard, or other meat sauce

Method:
1. Boil or broil wiener.
2. Place in a split wiener roll which has been heated.
3. Serve with mustard or other meat sauce of your choice.

Note: Your fat allowance may be used to butter the roll, if desired.

HOT DOG DELIGHT

Yield: 1 serving

Exchange for: 2 Meat Exchanges
and 1 Fat Exchange
and 2 Bread Exchanges

Ingredients: 1 wiener, cooked
1 slice pre-sliced processed cheese
1 strip partially cooked bacon
1 wiener roll

Method: 1. Roll cheese around wiener which has been cooked, and roll the partially cooked bacon around both cheese and wiener.

2. Fasten with a tooth pick.

3. Broil for 1 to 2 minutes.

4. Place on a heated wiener bun.

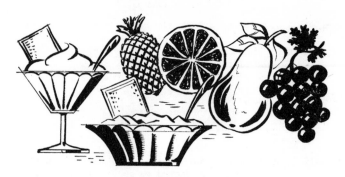

DESSERTS

"The mission of dessert is being that of a comforter of the stomach which being already appeased, nevertheless requires a little reflex flattery."

Desserts have many functions. There is the satisfaction that most people feel in having an attractive sweet at the end of a meal. They also supply nutrients required by a diet. For those who are on dietary restrictions, such as diabetics, there must be careful planning and use. Sweets, as such, do contain high percentages of sugar, so substitutions may have to be made.

Desserts fall into several categories. Fruit is abundantly available. Fresh fruit is often preferred and it can be used any time according to dietary allowances. Other desserts suitable for diabetics include gelatin whips in which fruits are used, and simple milk puddings which may be garnished with some fruit.

Many of these dessert recipes are also suitable for members of the family who are not diabetic.

DESSERTS, Classified According to Exchanges:

A — Milk Exchanges

1. Cocoa Floating Island
2. Apple Mousse
3. Soft Custard
4. Blanc Mange (Cream Pudding)
5. Junket
6. Baked Custard
7. Tapioca Pudding
8. Rice Pudding

B — Fruit Exchanges

1. Pumpkin Custard
2. Apple Snow
3. Apricot Whip
4. Banana Sponge
5. Jellied Fruits
6. Lime Fluff
7. Baked Apple
8. Chocolate Pudding

C — Combined Exchanges

1. Orange Pudding
2. Floating Island
3. Rice Pineapple Dessert
4. Graham Wafer Lemon Tart
5. Plum Pudding Recipe I
6. Plum Pudding Recipe II
7. Tarts
8. Shortcake
9. Dutch Apple Cake
10. Ice Cream Jelly Bavarian

D — Low Calorie

1. Orange Whip
2. Mocha Fluff
3. Coffee Jelly

Sauces

1. Chocolate Sauce
2. Lemon Sauce
3. Orange Sauce

A — Milk Exchanges

When using desserts which are calculated as a Milk Exchange, the fruit allowance for the meal may be used as fruit juice. If milk other than whole milk is used, make exchange for fat as suggested in the pages of general information.

COCOA FLOATING ISLAND

Yield: 6 servings

Exchange 1 serving for: $\frac{1}{4}$ Milk Exchange

Ingredients: 2 cups skim milk or reconstituted nonfat dry milk
3 eggs, separated
$\frac{1}{8}$ tsp. salt
$\frac{1}{2}$ tsp. vanilla
1 tsp. artificial liquid sweetener
2 tbsps. cocoa

Method: 1. Scald milk.
2. Put egg yolks in the top of a double boiler and beat lightly with a fork; add salt.
3. While stirring, gradually add the hot milk. Place over hot water.
4. Cook, stirring constantly, until the mixture thickens and forms a coating on a silver spoon.
5. Add vanilla and one half of the artificial liquid sweetener.
6. Strain and cool.
7. When ready to serve, beat egg whites until stiff.
8. Add cocoa and other half artificial liquid sweetener.
9. Place a heaping spoonful of this meringue on top of each serving of pudding.

APPLE MOUSSE

Yield: 6 servings

Exchange 1 serving for: ¼ Milk Exchange
and ½ Fruit Exchange

Ingredients: ¾ cup evaporated milk, thoroughly chilled
1½ cups unsweetened apple sauce
1½ tsps. lemon juice
⅜ tsp. salt
⅜ tsp. nutmeg
1½ tsps. artificial liquid sweetener

Method:
1. Whip evaporated milk until stiff. (Do not overwhip)
2. Fold in remaining ingredients.
3. Pour into individual molds, or into a tray, and freeze until firm.
4. Unmold, or cut if in a tray, and serve.

BLANC MANGE (CREAM PUDDING)

Yield: 6 servings

Exchange 1 serving for: ½ Milk Exchange
and 1 Fat Exchange

Ingredients: 2 tbsps. unflavored gelatin
6 tbsps. cold water
2¼ cups milk
¾ cup cream (18%)
6 cloves, whole
⅛ tsp. salt
¾ tsp. cinnamon
¾ tsp. vanilla
1½ tsps. artificial liquid sweetener

Method:
1. Add gelatin to cold water.
2. Boil cloves and cinnamon in ¼ cup hot water for 1 minute.
3. Strain into soaked gelatin — if this is not sufficient to dissolve the gelatin, heat in double boiler over hot water until dissolved.
4. Add milk and cream to dissolved gelatin.
5. Add vanilla, salt and artificial liquid sweetener.
6. Pour into six serving dishes; chill.

Note: May be unmolded and served with either fresh or canned fruit or a fruit sauce, which must be counted as a Fruit Exchange.

SOFT CUSTARD

Yield: 6 servings

Exchange 1 serving (1/3 cup) for: $\frac{1}{4}$ Milk Exchange

Ingredients: 2 cups milk
3 egg yolks
$\frac{1}{8}$ tsp. salt
$\frac{1}{2}$ tsp. vanilla
1 tsp. artificial liquid sweetener

Method:
1. Scald milk.
2. Place egg yolks in the top of a double boiler and beat slightly with a fork.
3. Add salt.
4. While stirring constantly, add hot milk gradually and cook over hot water until mixture forms a coating on a silver spoon.
5. Add vanilla and artificial liquid sweetener.
6. Strain and cool.

BAKED CUSTARD

Yield: 6 servings

Exchange 1 serving for: $\frac{1}{2}$ Milk Exchange

Ingredients: 2 cups milk
2 eggs
$\frac{1}{4}$ tsp. salt
$1\frac{1}{2}$ tsps. artificial liquid sweetener
1 tsp. vanilla
sprinkling of nutmeg

Method:
1. Scald milk.
2. Beat eggs slightly, add salt; add slowly to scalded milk.
3. Add artificial liquid sweetener and vanilla.
4. Strain and pour into 6 custard cups. Sprinkle with nutmeg.
5. Set cups in a shallow pan of hot water and oven poach for about 45 minutes in slow oven (325°F). Silver knife inserted into custard comes out clean when custard is done.

RICE PUDDING

Yield: 6 servings

Exchange 1 serving for: 1/4 Milk Exchange

Ingredients: 2 eggs
1 1/2 cups milk
pinch of salt
6 tbsps. cooked rice
1/8 tsp. vanilla
2 tsps. artificial liquid sweetener

Method: 1. Beat eggs.
2. Add milk, salt, artificial liquid sweetener, and vanilla to beaten eggs and mix.
3. Pour into 6 individual baking dishes and into each put 1 tbsp. of cooked rice.
4. Place baking dishes in a shallow pan of hot water.
5. Oven poach in a slow oven, 300°F, until set.

JUNKET

Yield: 4 servings

Exchange 1 serving for: 1/2 Milk Exchange

Ingredients: 1 junket tablet
1 tbsp. cold water
2 cups milk
1 tsp. artificial liquid sweetener
1 tsp. vanilla

Method: 1. Dissolve junket tablet in cold water.
2. Add sweetener.
3. Heat milk to lukewarm, remove from heat.
4. Add dissolved junket tablet and vanilla and stir quickly for a few seconds.
5. Pour immediately into individual serving dishes.
6. Allow to stand until firm. Chill.

TAPIOCA PUDDING

Yield: 4 servings
Exchange 1 serving for: ½ Milk Exchange
Ingredients: 2 eggs, separated
2 cups milk
3 tbsps. quick cooking tapioca
⅛ tsp. salt
½ tsp. vanilla
1 tsp. artificial liquid sweetener
Method: 1. Mix egg yolk with a small amount of milk in a saucepan.
2. Add remaining milk, tapioca and salt.
3. Cook over medium heat, stirring frequently until tapioca is transparent and mixture thickens slightly.
4. Remove from heat.
5. Add vanilla and artificial liquid sweetener.
6. Beat egg whites until they stand in soft peaks; add to tapioca mixture. Chill.

B — Fruit Exchanges

PUMPKIN CUSTARD

Yield: 6 servings
Exchange 1 serving for: ½ Fruit Exchange
Ingredients: ¾ cup canned pumpkin
¾ cup skim milk or reconstituted nonfat dry milk
1 egg
1 tsp. artificial liquid sweetener
¼ tsp. vanilla
½ tsp. cinnamon
¼ tsp. ginger
⅛ tsp. salt
Method: 1. Beat egg; add milk, vanilla, artificial liquid sweetener, salt, cinnamon, and ginger and mix.
2. Pour this mixture into the pumpkin which has been placed in a large bowl.
3. Mix well.
4. Pour into 6 custard cups; place cups in a pan with 1″ of hot water in it.
5. Oven poach in moderate oven (350°F) for 50 to 60 minutes, or until a silver knife, when inserted near the center of the custard, comes out clean.
Note: 1 tbsp. whipped cream (add 1 Fat Exchange) may be used as a garnish.

APPLE SNOW

Yield: 4 servings

Exchange 1 serving for: ½ Fruit Exchange

Ingredients: ½ tbsp. unflavored gelatin
⅛ tsp. salt
⅛ cup cold water
¼ cup boiling water
¼ tsp. grated lemon rind
½ tbsp. lemon juice
½ tsp. artificial liquid sweetener
⅞ cup artificially sweetened applesauce
2 egg whites

Method:
1. Mix gelatin and salt; add cold water to gelatin mixture.
2. Mix and let stand for 5 minutes.
3. Add boiling water to the gelatin mixture; stir until dissolved.
4. Add grated lemon rind, lemon juice, and applesauce.
5. Mix well. Sweeten with artificial sweetener.
6. Chill until partially set.
7. Beat egg whites until stiff, fold into gelatin mixture.
8. Pile into serving dishes. Chill.

BANANA SPONGE

Yield: 6 servings

Exchange 1 serving for: 1 Fruit Exchange

Ingredients: 1 tbsp. unflavored gelatin
¼ cup cold water
1/3 cup boiling water
½ tbsp. artificial liquid sweetener
2 tbsps. lemon juice
2/3 cup banana pulp
2 eggs whites

Method:
1. Soften gelatin in cold water.
2. Add artificial liquid sweetener to boiling water, and pour over softened gelatin, stirring until dissolved.
3. Add lemon juice.
4. Chill. Stir occasionally.
5. When partially set, add banana pulp; beat until foamy.
6. Add stiffly beaten egg whites and continue beating until mixture begins to stiffen.
7. Pile lightly in equal amounts into six serving dishes.

Note: May be served with 1 tbsp. whipped cream (add 1 Fat Exchange).

APRICOT WHIP

Yield: 6 servings

Exchange 1 serving for: 1 Fruit Exchange

Ingredients: ¾ cup unsweetened apricot pulp
¾ cup unsweetened apricot juice and water
1 tbsp. unflavored gelatin
1½ tsps. artificial liquid sweetener
1 tbsp. lemon juice
3 egg whites

Method: 1. Drain juice from apricots. Save juice.
2. Soften gelatin in part of the cold apricot juice and water.
3. Add softened gelatin to apricot pulp and the rest of the juice and water.
4. Heat over boiling water until gelatin is dissolved.
5. Add artificial sweetener and lemon juice.
6. Chill until partially set.
7. Beat egg whites until stiff; fold fruit mixture into beaten egg whites.
8. Pile into serving dishes. Chill.

Note: Prunes may be used instead of apricots to make Prune Whip; use ¾ cup prune pulp.

¾ cup banana pulp may be used to replace ¾ cup apricot pulp for Banana Whip.

LOW CALORIE DESSERTS
COFFEE JELLY

Yield: 2 servings

Exchange 1 serving for: May be eaten in this quantity without counting.

Ingredients: 2 tsps. unflavored gelatin
2 tbsps. cold water
1 cup hot, strong coffee
1 tbsp. artificial liquid sweetener
dash of salt

Method: 1. Soften gelatin in cold water.
2. Add hot, freshly made coffee, artificial liquid sweetener, and salt; stir until dissolved.
3. Pour into 2 molds. Chill until set.

Note: May be garnished with 1 tbsp. whipped cream (add 1 Fat Exchange).

JELLIED FRUITS

For a jellied fruit dessert, you may use any fruit or combination of fruits in amounts as allowed on the diet, or combined with an artificially sweetened jelly powder of your choice.

To allow for a fruit juice cocktail, use artificially sweetened jelly powder as a dessert with $1/2$ Fruit Exchange in fruit and use other $1/2$ Fruit Exchange in fruit juice to make up a fruit juice cocktail by adding artificially sweetened gingerale; e.g. orange jelly with 1/3 cup fruit cocktail; and $1/4$ cup grapefruit juice with artificially sweetened gingerale.

Note: You may use 1 tbsp. whipped cream (add 1 Fat Exchange) as a garnish **OR** you may use 1 serving of soft custard $1/2$ Milk Exchange) with the jellied fruit.

LIME FLUFF

Yield: 8 servings

Exchange 1 serving for: $1/2$ Fruit Exchange

Ingredients: 1 tbsp. artificially sweetened lime jelly powder
$3/4$ cup boiling water
$5/8$ cup unsweetened applesauce
6 ozs. evaporated milk (very cold)
1 tbsp. lemon juice
1 tsp. artificial liquid sweetener

Method:
1. Dissolve jelly powder in boiling water.
2. Add applesauce and artificial liquid sweetener. Mix well.
3. Cool until partially thickened.
4. Add lemon juice to evaporated milk and whip until stiff.
5. Add whipped milk to partially set jelly and applesauce mixture and beat slowly until mixed.
6. Pour into 8 serving dishes and chill.
7. May garnish with fruit from Fruit Exchange.

BAKED APPLE

Yield: 1 serving

Exchange for: 1 Fruit Exchange

Ingredients: 1 small-sized apple
1 tsp. orange juice
few grains of cinnamon or nutmeg

Method:
1. Core apple. Score skin to prevent bursting.
2. Place in baking dish. Sprinkle with cinnamon or nutmeg. Add orange juice and 3 tbsps. water.
3. Bake in moderate oven, (350°F) about 1 hour.

CHOCOLATE PUDDING

Yield: 6 servings
Exchange 1 serving for: ½ Fruit Exchange
Ingredients: 6 tbsps. cold water
3 tsps. unflavored gelatin
2 cups skim milk or reconstituted nonfat dry milk
salt and cinnamon to flavor
few drops vanilla
8 tsps. cocoa
1 tbsp. artificial liquid sweetener
Method: 1. Soak gelatin in cold water.
2. Mix cocoa, artificial liquid sweetener, salt, vanilla, and cinnamon; add to hot milk.
3. Heat milk mixture and add to gelatin mixture.
4. Stir until gelatin is dissolved.
5. Pour into molds and allow to set.

C — Combined Exchanges
ORANGE PUDDING

Yield: 6 servings
Exchange 1 serving for: 1 Fruit Exchange
and 1 Meat Exchange
Ingredients: 2 cups whole milk
grated rind from 1 orange
3 tbsps. cornstarch
1 tsp. artificial liquid sweetener
½ cup cold milk
pinch of salt
3 egg yolks
1 tsp. vanilla
3 egg whites
Method: 1. Scald 2 cups milk and orange rind.
2. Mix cornstarch, salt, artificial liquid sweetener, and ½ cup cold milk.
3. Add to the hot milk.
4. Stir and cook over boiling water until fully thickened.
5. Cover and cook about 30 minutes.
6. Add the beaten egg yolks and vanilla; mix well and cook for another 2 or 3 minutes.
7. Pour into a baking dish.
8. Cover with egg whites which have been beaten until stiff.
9. Bake in slow oven (300°F) just until egg whites are lightly browned.

FLOATING ISLAND

Yield: 6 servings
Exchange 1 serving for: 1 Meat Exchange
and ½ Milk Exchange
Ingredients: 3 cups milk
6 egg yolks
1 tsp. artificial liquid sweetener
¾ tsp. vanilla
6 egg whites, beaten stiff
Method:
1. Make a soft custard of first four ingredients. (See page 95 — desserts)
2. Pour into six serving dishes.
3. To stiffly beaten egg whites, add a few drops of vanilla and 1 tsp. artificial liquid sweetener.
4. Make 6 mounds of this meringue in baking dish. Bake in moderate oven (350°F) until a golden brown.
5. Place a browned meringue on top of each serving of custard.

RICE PINEAPPLE DESSERT

Yield: 6 servings
Exchange 1 serving for: ½ Milk Exchange
and 1 Fruit Exchange
and 1 Fat Exchange (See below)
Ingredients: 1⅛ cups evaporated milk
1 tbsp. lemon juice
1½ tbsps. unflavored gelatin
1½ cups cooked rice
¾ cup unsweetened crushed pineapple, drained
1½ tsps. artificial liquid sweetener
dash of salt
⅜ cup whipped cream, if fat allowance is sufficient
Method:
1. Chill ¾ cup evaporated milk.
2. Soften gelatin in remaining amount of milk and dissolve over hot water.
3. Add dissolved gelatin to cooked rice.
4. Add pineapple, artificial liquid sweetener, and salt.
5. Add lemon juice to evaporated milk.
6. Whip chilled evaporated milk stiff, and fold into rice mixture.
7. Serve with a topping of whipped cream, if allowed.
Note: ¾ cup unsweetened diced apricots may be used in place of the pineapple.

GRAHAM WAFER LEMON TART

Yield: 6 servings

Exchange 1 tart shell for: ½ Bread Exchange
and 1 Fat Exchange

Exchange 1 serving of filling for: Free Food, List A

Ingredients: Crust:
12 graham wafers
2 tbsps. butter or margarine
1 tsp. artificial liquid sweetener
dash of cinnamon
Filling:
6 tbsps. artificially sweetened lemon jelly powder
3 cups water
3 egg whites
1½ tsps. grated lemon rind
few drops lemon juice

Method:
1. Crush graham wafers.
2. Melt butter or margarine; add to crushed graham wafers, artificial liquid sweetener, and cinnamon.
3. Press into 6 tart shells; bake in moderate oven (325°F) for 5 minutes. Chill before removing from pan.
4. Make up jelly powder as directed on package.
5. Chill until slightly thickened; beat until fluffy with an egg beater.
6. Beat egg whites until stiff.
7. Fold in grated lemon rind, lemon juice, and beaten egg whites.
8. Fill tart shells with filling. Chill.

Note: Extra filling (Free Food, List A) may be used as pudding.

SHORTCAKE

Use: 1 serving of Orange Cake (See page 110) or 1 tea biscuit (See page 114) and exchange for 1 Bread Exchange and 1 or 1½ Fat Exchange. Use allowance of fruit for meal. You may garnish the shortcake with 1 tbsp. whipped cream (add 1 Fat Exchange).

PLUM PUDDING RECIPE #1

Yield: 4 servings

Exchange 1 serving for: 1 Fruit Exchange
and ½ Bread Exchange

Ingredients: 1 tbsp. artificially sweetened orange jelly powder
1 cup boiling water
¼ cup Grapenuts
4 canned, artificially sweetened plums, chopped fine
4 tbsps. raisins, chopped fine
1/8 tsp. nutmeg
pinch of cloves and cinnamon

Method:
1. Mix nutmeg, cinnamon and cloves with the jelly powder.
2. Add boiling water and stir until the jelly powder is dissolved.
3. Cool. When jelly is partially set, add the chopped plums, chopped raisins and the Grapenuts.
4. Mix well.
5. Place in refrigerator until set.
6. Unmould when ready to serve.

Note: 1 tbsp. whipped cream (add 1 Fat Exchange) may be used as a topping.

PLUM PUDDING RECIPE #2

Yield: 6 servings

Exchange 1 serving for: 1 Fruit Exchange
and 1 Fat Exchange

Ingredients: 9 tbsps. grated raw carrot
6 tbsps. raisins
6 tbsps. suet
6 egg yolks
6 tbsps. flour
6 tsps. grated lemon rind
1 tbsp. artificial liquid sweetener
¾ tsp. allspice
¾ tsp. nutmeg
¾ tsp. cinnamon
¾ tsp. vanilla
few grains salt

Method:
1. Mix all ingredients together.
2. Divide into 6 individual molds and steam 30 to 40 minutes.

TARTS

Yield: 12 small tart shells

Exchange 1 tart shell for: 1 Bread Exchange
and 1 Fat Exchange

Ingredients: 1½ cups sifted flour
½ cup shortening
½ tsp. salt
3 tbsps. ice water

Method:
1. Mix flour and salt.
2. Cut shortening into flour mixture.
3. Sprinkle in ice water and mix.
4. Roll out on a lightly floured board.
5. Line 12 tart shell pans with pastry. Bake in hot oven (400°F)

FILLING FOR TARTS

Fruit — Use allowance of fruit for meal.

Pumpkin — Use Pumpkin Custard Filling — ½ Fruit Exchange.

Lemon — Use recipe for Graham Wafer Lemon Tart Filling.

ICE CREAM JELLY BAVARIAN

Yield: 6 servings

Exchange 1 serving for: 1 Fruit Exchange
and 1 Fat Exchange

Ingredients: 2 tbsps. artificially sweetened jelly powder (orange, strawberry, lime, etc.)
2 cups boiling water
1 pint brick of ice cream (or 6 ice cream rolls)

Method:
1. Dissolve the jelly powder in boiling water.
2. Allow to cool slightly.
3. Remove ice cream from the freezer and leave at room temperature for 5 minutes. Cut into small pieces for easier handling.
4. Using a rotary beater or an electric mixer at slow speed, add ice cream, one piece at a time, mixing until ice cream is melted.
5. Pour into serving dishes, dividing evenly into 6 servings. Chill.
6. May be unmolded for serving, if desired.

DUTCH APPLE CAKE

Yield: 6 servings

Exchange 1 serving for: 1 Fruit Exchange
and 1 Bread Exchange
and 1 Fat Exchange

Ingredients: 1½ cups flour
½ tsp. salt
3 tsps. baking powder
2 tbsps. shortening
¼ cup water
¼ cup skim milk or reconstituted nonfat dry milk
1 tbsp. artificial liquid sweetener
2 medium-sized apples
1 tsp. cinnamon

Method:
1. Sift flour, salt, and baking powder.
2. Cut shortening into flour.
3. Add milk, water and artificial liquid sweetener.
4. Mix well.
5. Spread dough to about ½-inch thickness on greased pan.
6. Wash, pare, core and slice apples.
7. Place apples on dough in rows, putting sharp edges into dough.
8. Sprinkle with cinnamon.
9. Bake in moderate oven (350°F) 30 to 40 minutes. Serve hot.

ORANGE WHIP

Yield: 6 servings

Exchange 1 serving for: 1 Fruit Exchange List 3

Ingredients: 6 tbsps. artificially sweetened orange jelly powder
¾ cup boiling water
¾ cup orange juice
12 ozs. artificially sweetened gingerale
3 egg whites

Method:
1. Dissolve jelly powder in boiling water.
2. Add orange juice, gingerale, and chill.
3. When partially set, whip until foamy.
4. Fold in beaten egg whites.
5. Pile lightly into 6 serving dishes. Chill.

MOCHA FLUFF

Yield: 6 servings

Exchange 1 serving for: May be used in this amount without counting.

Ingredients: 1½ tbsps. unflavored gelatin
⅜ cup cold water
1½ tsps. artificial liquid sweetener
2 cups hot, strong coffee
3 tbsps. lemon juice
3 egg whites

Method: 1. Soften gelatin in cold water.
2. Add artificial liquid sweetener, hot coffee and stir until thoroughly dissolved.
3. Add lemon juice. Cool.
4. When nearly set, beat until mixture thickens.
5. Add stiffly beaten egg whites and continue beating until the mixture holds its shape.
6. Pile into 6 individual serving dishes.

Note: May use 1 tbsp. whipped cream (add 1 Fat Exchange) to garnish dessert.

Sauces for Desserts

CHOCOLATE SAUCE

Yield: 1 cup

Exchange 1 tbsp. sauce for: 1 Bread Exchange List 4

Ingredients: 1 tbsp. butter or margarine
3 tbsps. cocoa
1 tbsp. cornstarch
few grains salt
1 cup skim milk or reconstituted nonfat dry milk
1 tbsp. artificial liquid sweetener
½ tsp. vanilla

Method: 1. Melt butter or margarine.
2. Combine cocoa, cornstarch and salt and blend with melted butter or margarine until smooth.
3. Add milk and artificial liquid sweetener and cook over moderate heat, stirring constantly until slightly thickened, and there is no taste of raw starch.
4. Remove from the heat; stir in vanilla.
5. Set pan in ice water and stir until completely cool. (Sauce thickens as it cools.)

ORANGE SAUCE (For Plum Pudding Recipe #2)

Yield: 1 cup sauce

Exchange 2 tbsps. sauce for: ¼ Bread Exchange List 4

Ingredients: 1 cup water
¼ tsp. grated orange rind
few drops lemon juice
1 tsp. artificial liquid sweetener
4 tsps. cornstarch
4 tbsps. orange juice

Method:
1. Mix ¼ cup of water with the cornstarch.
2. To remaining water, add the orange rind.
3. Mix together and cook until clear (about 1 or 2 minutes) and there is no taste of raw starch.
4. Add lemon and orange juices and artificial liquid sweetener.
5. Serve warm.

LEMON SAUCE

Yield: 1 cup

Exchange 2 tbsps. sauce for: ¼ Bread Exchange List 4

Ingredients: 1 tbsp. cornstarch
⅛ tsp. salt
2 tbsps. cold water
1 cup boiling water
2 tsps. butter or margarine
1 tbsp. grated lemon rind
2 tsps. artificial liquid sweetener
2 tbsps. lemon juice

Method:
1. Combine cornstarch and salt and blend with cold water and artificial liquid sweetener.
2. Add boiling water gradually, stirring constantly.
3. Continue stirring and cook over medium heat until mixture clears (about 1 or 2 minutes) and there is no taste of raw starch.
4. Remove from heat; add lemon juice, lemon rind and butter; mix well.

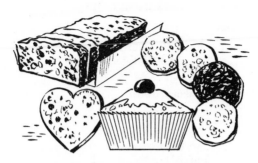

CAKES, COOKIES
AND QUICK BREADS

An anniversary perhaps? Company for dinner? Or just a family affair? There's something for every occasion.

For a special treat, try any of the following recipes, but take a tip from us — Do follow the recipes exactly, and remember that all measurements are level.

CUP CAKE RECIPE

Yield: 15 cup cakes

Exchange 1 cup cake for: 1 Bread Exchange
and 1 Fat Exchange

Ingredients: 1½ cups sifted flour
½ tsp. salt
4 tsps. baking powder
2 tsps. artificial liquid sweetener
2 eggs, well beaten
¼ cup milk
4 tbsps. melted vegetable shortening or vegetable oil

Method: 1. Sift flour, salt and baking powder together.
2. Combine remaining ingredients with sifted mixture.
3. Stir only until dry ingredients are moistened. (Batter will be lumpy.)

Note: 40 grams uncooked batter will give 30 grams cooked batter.

For Shortcake — use 4 tbsps. melted butter or margarine instead of shortening and add ½ tsp. vanilla.

For Pudding — serve with fruit allowance as an Upside-Down Pudding.

ORANGE CAKE

Yield: 10 servings

Exchange 1 serving for: 1 Bread Exchange
and 1½ Fat Exchanges

Ingredients: 1 cup sifted flour
1½ tsps. baking powder
½ tsp. salt
¼ cup vegetable oil
3 egg yolks
½ cup unsweetened frozen orange juice concentrate
1 tbsp. artificial liquid sweetener
3 egg whites
¼ tsp. cream of tartar
1 tsp. grated orange rind

Method:
1. Mix and sift dry ingredients thoroughly several times.
2. Make a well in the mixture.
3. Add in order: vegetable oil, unbeaten egg yolks, orange juice concentrate, and artificial liquid sweetener. Beat until smooth.
4. Place egg whites in a bowl.
5. Add cream of tartar and beat until very stiff.
6. Fold stiffly beaten egg whites and grated orange rind into the flour mixture.
7. Pour into 9" tube pan, and bake in moderate oven (325°F) 35 minutes or until it tests done.

COMMERCIAL CAKE MIXES

Chocolate Cake:— Make in 8" square pan, according to directions on package. The cake is cut 4 x 5, yielding 20 servings.
The Exchange for 1 serving is: 1 Bread Exchange
and 1 Fat Exchange

White Cake:— Make in 8" square pan, according to directions on package. The cake is cut 4 x 5, yielding 20 servings.
The Exchange for 1 serving is: 1 Bread Exchange
and 1 Fat Exchange

Angel Cake Mix:— Make in angel cake pan according to directions on package. Large cake mix is cut into 20 servings. Small cake mix is cut into 10 servings.
The Exchange for 1 serving is: 1 Bread Exchange

CINNAMON SPICE COOKIES

Yield: 30 cookies

Exchange 4 cookies for: 1 Fruit Exchange
and 1 Fat Exchange

Ingredients: 5 tbsps. butter or margarine
1 cup sifted flour
½ tsp. baking powder
pinch of salt
2 tsps. artificial liquid sweetener
1 tsp. vanilla
1 tbsp. milk, or fruit juice, or coffee
1 tsp. cinnamon

Method:
1. Cream butter or margarine until light and fluffy.
2. Blend in sifted flour, baking powder, cinnamon and salt.
3. Mix artificial liquid sweetener with vanilla and milk or other liquid.
4. Stir into flour mixture and mix thoroughly.
5. Shape dough into 30 even-sized balls, and place on a cookie sheet.
6. Flatten balls with a fork dipped in cold water.
7. Bake 10 to 15 minutes in moderate oven (375°F)

COCONUT FLUFFS

Yield: 12 fluffs

Exchange 1 fluff for: 1 Fat Exchange

Ingredients: 6 level tbsps. cream cheese
1 tsp. artificial liquid sweetener
½ tsp. mixed grated orange and lemon rind
1 tsp. chopped almonds or walnuts
¼ cup shredded coconut

Method:
1. Toast the coconut in oven until lightly brown.
2. With spoon, mix cheese and artificial liquid sweetener until light and fluffy.
3. Add grated rind and nuts to the cheese, and mix thoroughly.
4. Form into 12 balls. Roll in toasted coconut
5. Refrigerate until serving time.

Variation: Instead of toasting the coconut it might be colored with a sugarless food coloring.

BROWNIES

Yield: 16 cookies
Exchange 1 cookie for: 1 Fruit Exchange
and 1 Fat Exchange
Ingredients: 2 cups fine graham cracker crumbs (24 crackers)
½ cup chopped walnuts
3 ozs. semi-sweet chocolate pieces
2 tsps. artificial liquid sweetener
¼ tsp. salt
1 cup skim milk or reconstituted nonfat dry milk
Method: 1. Preheat oven to moderate (350°F).
2. Place all ingredients in a bowl and stir until blended.
3. Turn into slightly greased pan 8″ x 8″ x 2″. Bake 30 minutes at 350°F.
4. Cut into 16 two-inch squares while warm.

CHEESE MOONS

Yield: 32 cookies
Exchange 1 cookie for: 1 Fruit Exchange
and 2 Fat Exchanges
Ingredients: ½ lb. butter or margarine
½ lb. cream cheese
2 cups sifted cake flour
artificially sweetened jam spread
Method: 1. Mix butter or margarine and cream cheese together.
2. Add flour slowly, reserving some to flour the baking board. When the dough becomes stiff, turn it out on the floured board and knead in the remaining flour, working with hands. Roll thin.
3. Cut with round cutter into 32 cookies.
4. Place ½ to 1 tsp. jam spread on one half of each cookie.
5. Fold over and press edges together.
6. Bake in moderate oven (350°F to 375°F) until golden brown.

FRUIT BALLS

Yield: 18 fruit balls
Exchange 1 fruit ball for: ½ Fruit Exchange
and ½ Fat Exchange
Ingredients: ½ cup chopped dates
½ cup chopped walnuts
½ cup artificially sweetened canned red cherries

Method: 1. Mix fruit and nuts.
2. Add just enough cherry juice to hold together.
3. Form into balls (allowing about 1½ tbsps. per fruit ball.)

They may be rolled in: (1) Coconut , allowing 1 tsp. shredded cocoanut per fruit ball; (2) finely chopped walnuts, allowing 1 tsp. per fruit ball; (3) artificially sweetened vanilla pudding powder. In these amounts, none of these additions will appreciably change the food value of the cookies.

NUT COOKIES

Yield: 36 cookies

Exchange 1 cookie for: ½ Fat Exchange

Exchange 2 cookies for: ½ Fruit Exchange
and 1 Fat Exchange

Ingredients: 1/3 cup butter or margarine
1½ tsps. artificial liquid sweetener
2 tbsps. orange juice
1 tsp. grated orange rind
1 cup sifted flour
¼ tsp. baking powder
½ tsp. salt
½ cup chopped walnuts
½ tsp. vanilla

Method: 1. Cream butter or margarine with artificial liquid sweetener; add orange juice and orange rind.
2. Sift flour, baking powder and salt together; add chopped nuts and mix until the nuts are covered with the flour mixture.
3. Add the sifted flour, nuts, and vanilla to the butter mixture and mix well together.
4. Form into a long narrow roll; wrap in waxed paper and chill in the refrigerator until very firm.
5. Slice very thin into 36 cookies.
6. Bake in moderate oven (375°F) about 12 minutes, or until lightly browned.

CORNFLAKE CRISPS

Yield: 20 cookies
Exchange 1 cookie for: 1 Bread Exchange List 4
Ingredients: ¼ cup oats
1 egg white
⅛ tsp. salt
1 tsp. artificial liquid sweetener
¼ tsp. vanilla
¾ cup cornflakes
Method: 1. Oven-toast the oats until the flakes are golden brown.
2. Add salt to egg white and beat until stiff, but not dry.
3. Beating continually, add vanilla and artificial liquid sweetener.
4. Fold in the cornflakes and toasted oats.
5. Drop by spoonful on slightly greased baking sheet.
6. Bake in slow oven (325°F) 15 to 20 minutes.

TASTY COOKIES

Yield: 19 cookies
Exchange 2 cookies for: 1 Bread Exchange
Ingredients: ½ cup flour
¼ tsp. salt
3 tbsps. shortening
1 tbsp. milk
1 tsp. artificial liquid sweetener
½ cup quick oats
¼ tsp. baking soda
Method: 1. Mix all dry ingredients together, then rub in shortening.
2. Mix to stiff dough with very little milk.
3. Roll out very, very thinly; cut into 19 rounds with a cookie cutter.
4. Bake on slightly greased cookie sheet for 20 to 25 minutes in slow oven (325°F) until lightly browned.

TEA BISCUITS

Yield: 10 biscuits of equal size
Exchange 1 biscuit for: 1 Bread Exchange
and 1 Fat Exchange
Ingredients: 2 cups sifted flour
4 tsps. baking powder
½ tsp. salt
3 tbsps. fat (reserve some to grease the pan)
2/3 cup skim milk

Method: 1. Sift flour, baking powder, and salt.
2. Cut in the fat with a knife until very fine.
3. Pour in milk, stir with a fork until mixed.
4. Turn out on slightly floured board. Knead lightly, and roll ¾" thick.
5. Cut with a knife into 10 biscuits of equal size.
6. Place on slightly greased pan.
7. Bake in hot oven (400°F to 425°F) for 15 to 20 minutes.

SCOTCH OATCAKES #1

Yield: 24 cookies
Exchange 1 cookie for: ½ Bread Exchange
and 1 Fat Exchange
Ingredients: 1 cup sifted flour
2 cups quick oats
¼ tsp. salt
½ cup shortening
¼ cup milk
⅜ tsp. artificial liquid sweetener
Method: 1. Mix flour, oatmeal, and salt.
2. Add melted shortening and mix well; then add milk to which artificial liquid sweetener has been added.
3. Roll out on slightly floured board.
4. Cut into 24 cookies.
5. Bake on slightly greased cookie sheet in moderate oven (350°F to 375°F) until golden brown.

SCOTCH OATCAKES #2

Yield: 24 cookies
Exchange 1 cookie for: 1 Fruit Exchange
and 1 Fat Exchange
Ingredients: 1/3 cup shortening
4 cups oats
¼ tsp. salt
Method: 1. Mix oats and shortening.
2. Roll thin on slightly floured board.
3. Cut into 24 cookies.
4. Bake on slightly greased cookie sheet in moderate oven (350°F to 375°F) until golden brown.
Variations: 1. Add 2 tbsps. chopped walnuts to the full recipe. The food value of the cookie is not changed appreciably.
2. Add 2 tbsps. shredded coconut to the full recipe. The food value of the cookie is not changed appreciably.

WAFFLES

Yield: About 30 waffles

Exchange 1 tbsp. mixture for: ½ Fruit Exchange or
1/3 Bread Exchange

Ingredients: 2 cups sifted flour
3 tsps. baking powder
½ tsp. salt
2 egg yolks
2 egg whites
1 2/3 cups skim milk or reconstituted nonfat dry milk
1½ tbsps. melted butter or margarine
¼ tsp. artificial liquid sweetener

Method:
1. Sift dry ingredients together.
2. Gradually add beaten egg yolks, milk, and butter or margarine and fold in stiffly beaten egg whites.
3. Heat waffle iron.
4. Pour 1 tbsp. mixture in each section near the center.
5. Bake until crisp and brown.
6. Serve at once with 1 tsp. artificially sweetened jam spread.

BLUEBERRY MUFFINS

Yield: 12 muffins

Exchange 1 muffin for: 1 Bread Exchange
and 1 Fat Exchange

Ingredients: 2 cups sifted flour
2½ tsps. baking powder
1 tsp. salt
½ cup blueberries
1 egg, beaten lightly
2 tsps. artificial liquid sweetener
1 cup milk
2 tbsps. melted butter or margarine

Method:
1. Sift the flour again with baking powder and salt.
2. Add the blueberries to the flour mixture and mix until well coated.
3. Add egg, milk, and melted butter or margarine; mix until blended.
4. Divide batter evenly into 12 lightly greased muffin tins.
5. Bake in moderate oven (375°F) 20 to 30 minutes.

ORANGE NUT BREAD

Yield: 12 servings
Exchange 1 serving for: 1 Bread Exchange
and 1 Fat Exchange
Ingredients: 2 cups sifted flour
1½ tsps. baking powder
½ tsp. baking soda
¼ tsp. salt
1 egg
1/3 cup skim milk or reconstituted nonfat dry milk
2 tbsps. melted butter or margarine
1 tbsp. artificial liquid sweetener
½ cup artificially sweetened orange fruit spread
¼ cup chopped walnuts or pecans
Method: 1. Combine flour, baking powder, baking soda and salt in mixing bowl. Sift.
2. Beat egg; add skim milk and artificial liquid sweetener.
3. Add to flour mixture.
4. Stir only until all flour is dampened and gradually mix in the melted butter or margarine.
5. Fold in orange fruit spread and chopped nuts, mixing as little as possible.
6. Place in lightly greased 9" x 5" x 3" loaf pan.
7. Bake in moderate oven (350°F) for 1 hour and 40 minutes or until loaf springs back when pressed lightly with the finger.
8. Cool before slicing.

BRAN MUFFINS

Yield: 9 muffins
Exchange 1 muffin for: 1 Bread Exchange
Ingredients: ½ cup flour
½ tsp. baking soda
½ tsp. salt
1 cup prepared bran cereal
1 egg, beaten
¼ cup molasses
5/8 cup milk
Method: 1. Sift flour, soda, and salt together.
2. Add bran, eggs, and molasses.
3. Add milk and stir until dry ingredients are just dampened.
4. Grease 9 muffin tins very lightly.
5. Divide mixture into 9 equal portions.
6. Bake in moderate oven (375°F) 20 to 30 minutes.

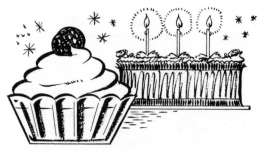

FROSTINGS AND TOPPINGS

To add a touch of glamor to cakes, cup cakes and some desserts!

FRUIT FROSTING

Yield: ¼ cup frosting

Exchange 1 tbsp. frosting for: 1 Fat Exchange

Ingredients: 4 tbsps. cream cheese
2 tsps. artificially sweetened jam spread (pineapple or strawberry)

Methor: 1. Soften cream cheese at room temperature for about ½ hour.
2. Add the jam spread and beat vigorously with rotary beater or electric mixer.
3. Spread on cake or cup cakes, allowing 1 tbsp. of frosting per serving.

Variations: 1. In place of the jam spread, mix ½ tsp. of instant coffee with 2 tsps. hot water, and add one ¼-grain tablet artificial sweetener and dissolve. Finish as above.
2. To the plain cream cheese, add 1 tbsp. milk, one ¼-grain tablet artificial sweetener dissolved in the milk, and 1 or 2 drops vanilla. Make as above.
3. Add unsweetened artificial coloring of choice to the plain frosting.
4. For orange icing, add ¼ tsp. grated orange rind to the plain frosting.
5. For lemon frosting, add ⅛ to ¼ tsp. grated lemon rind to the plain frosting.

CHOCOLATE FROSTING

Yield: 8 servings

Exchange ⅛ of this recipe for: ¼ Milk Exchange List 1

Ingredients: 1 oz. unsweetened chocolate
6 tbsps. evaporated milk
½ tsp. vanilla
1 tsp. (or more) artificial liquid sweetener

Method: 1. Melt chocolate over hot water.
2. Stir in evaporated milk.
3. Mix well and cook until it thickens, about 2 or 3 minutes.
4. Remove from heat and stir in vanilla and artificial liquid sweetener. If too thick for spreading, thin down to spreading consistency with water.

SKIM MILK TOPPING

Yield: 4 servings

Exchange 1 serving for: ⅛ cup skim milk

Ingredients: ¼ cup skim milk powder or crystals
¼ cup ice water
½ tsp. artificial liquid sweetener

Method: 1. Combine ingredients.
2. Beat on high speed of electric mixer or vigorously with rotary beater until consistency of whipped cream.

WHIPPED CREAM

Exchange 1 rounded tbsp. whipped cream, plain, or with any of the following additions for: 1 Fat Exchange

Variations: 1. Unsweetened artificial coloring may be added to whipped cream without changing the food value.
2. A drop of artificial liquid sweetener and a drop of vanilla may be added to the whipped cream without changing the food value.
3. ¼ tsp. instant coffee may be added to ¼ cup whipped cream before beating.

"FROSTICLE"

Exchange 1 "frosticle" for: 1 Foods as desired

Ingredients: 2 pkgs. flavoured artificially sweetened jelly powder
1 cup boiling water
2 cups cold water or artificially sweetened gingerale

Method: 1. Dissolve jelly powder in boiling water.
2. Add cold water or ginger ale.
3. Freeze in ice-cube tray or containers available in retail stores for this purpose.
Wooden sticks may be inserted into each when partially frozen.

PEANUT CRUSH

Yield: 6 servings

Exchange 1 serving for: 1 Fat Exchange
and ¼ Bread Exchange List 4

Ingredients: 2½ tbsps. peanut butter
2 tsps. artificially sweetened jam spread
4 graham wafers or social teas, crushed
10 peanuts, chopped fine
or 6 walnuts, chopped fine

Method: 1. Mix peanut butter, jam spread and crushed biscuits together.
2. Form into six balls. Roll in chopped nuts.

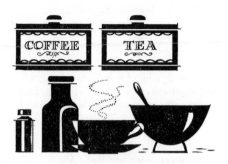

BEVERAGES

Tea and coffee, when served clear, are not counted in the Exchanges. Variations of these and other suggestions for beverages are included here to give some ideas for adding variety to meals. In many cases, variety is achieved with a minimum number of exchanges. As well, tempting fluids are a help in times of illness, providing easily assimilated nourishment.

Recipes and suggestions for soft and liquid diets are included in a separates section. (See pages 127-133)

HOT BEVERAGES

Coffee

Whether instant or ground coffee is used, is a matter of personal preference.

Instant coffee made in bulk, and served piping hot from a coffee pot or carafe, has good flavor

If coffee is to be brewed, choose the grind which suits your coffee maker. Buy coffee in small quantities to ensure freshness and store it in an air-tight container. Use a sparkling-clean coffee maker, and water at a rolling boil. Measure coffee and water exactly, and follow carefully the instructions for the type of coffee maker used. Brew just long enough to extract best flavor , remove immediately from grounds, and serve steaming hot.

Café Au Lait

Heat milk allowance just to scalding point in double boiler or over low heat. Combine with an equal amount of strong, hot coffee by pouring both into the cup at the same time. If desired, add artificial liquid sweetener to taste.

Spiced Coffee

Brew coffee as usual, adding a mixture of spices to the grounds. A pleasant combination of spices for 4 cups of coffee is: 4 whole cloves; $\frac{1}{8}$ tsp. nutmeg; $\frac{1}{8}$ tsp. cinnamon. Serve the coffee with cinnamon sticks as stirrers.

Tea

Bring fresh cold water to a rapid boil. Allow 1 tea bag or 1 heaping tsp. of tea leaves for each 2 teacups of water.

Heat the teapot (not metal) by pouring in a little boiling water. Empty the pot, immediately put in the measured tea, and add the freshly boiled water.

Let steep for 3 to 5 minutes. Stir, and serve at once.

For variety, experiment with green tea, oolong, or special blends.

Hot Spiced Tea: Stud lemon slices with whole cloves. Place 1 lemon slice in each tea cup, add a 1-inch stick of cinnamon, and pour in the hot tea.

COCOA

Yield: 1 serving

Exchange for: $\frac{1}{2}$ Milk Exchange
and $\frac{1}{2}$ Bread Exchange List 4

Ingredients: $\frac{1}{2}$ cup milk
2 teaspoons powdered cocoa (not instant)
artificial liquid sweetener to taste

Method: 1. Measure milk into a saucepan, and cocoa into a cup. Remove 1 tbsp. of the milk, and blend with the cocoa powder.
2. Scald remaining milk, adding artificial liquid sweetener. Gradually stir scalded milk into cocoa mixture.
3. Sprinkle with grated nutmeg if desired.

Note: If Fat Allowance permits, top with 1 rounded tbsp. whipped cream (add 1 Fat Exchange).

HOT SPICED APPLE JUICE

Yield: 4 servings (2/3 cup each)

Exchange 1 serving for: 2 Fruit Exchanges

Ingredients: 2 and 2/3 cups apple juice
½ tsp. whole allspice
6 whole cloves
1 two-inch stick cinnamon

Method: 1. Add spices to apple juice in saucepan; bring just to a boil.
2. Strain into heated glasses, and serve. Delightful on crisp fall days.

COLD BEVERAGES

Iced Coffee

Pour double-strength coffee over ice cubes or cracked ice in tall glasses. If the ice supply is limited, allow the coffee to cool first to room temperature (in which case, the coffee may be made a little less strong). If desired, add artificial liquid sweetener to taste.

Using 1 Fat Exchange, top with 1 rounded tbsp. of whipped cream, flavored with vanilla.

Iced Tea

Brew tea double-strength. Fill tall glasses with ice, and carefully pour in the tea. Some blends of tea are less likely than others to turn cloudy when poured over ice — e.g., certain blends of English Breakfast Tea.

Green and oolong teas are pleasant, but pale in colour, and are best suited for use with fruit juices in making punch.

Serve iced tea with a wedge of lemon and a sprig of mint, and with artificial liquid sweetener if desired.

TEA PUNCH

Yield: six 6-oz. servings

Exchange 1 serving for: 1 Fruit Exchange

Ingredients: 1 cup tea (made from 2 tsps. green or oolong tea and 1 cup water)
½ cup lemon juice
½ cup pineapple juice
1½ cups orange juice
1 cup water
artificial liquid sweetener to taste

Method: Combine all ingredients; chill, and serve over ice.

CRANBERRY PUNCH

Yield: ten 4-oz. servings

Exchange 1 serving for: 1/2 Fruit Exchange

Ingredients: 1 cup raw cranberries
1 1/2 cups water
3/4 cup lemon juice
1 1/4 cups orange juice
artificial liquid sweetener to taste
2 cups soda water

Method: 1. Sort and wash the cranberries. Put into a saucepan and add the water. Cover and cook until the skins pop.
2. Press the cranberries through a sieve; add fruit juices and sweeten to taste with artificial liquid sweetener. Chill.
3. At serving time, pour over ice and add the soda water.

QUICK PUNCH: Mix 1 Fruit Exchange, as juice, with artificially sweetened ginger ale or with soda water.

Serving Hint: When using a punch bowl, chill the punch with larger pieces of ice, made by freezing water in cans from frozen juices.

To carry out the colour scheme of a party, first tint the water for the ice with pure food coloring. Freeze mint leaves, tiny wedges of orange and lemon slices, or fresh berries or cherries in the ice.

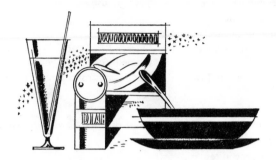

DIABETIC LIQUID
AND SOFT DIETS

The diabetic patient who is in the hospital faces no problem when the doctor orders a liquid or soft diet. However, when the diabetic is ill at home, adapting his daily meal plan to liquid or soft foods often causes bewilderment and consternation. The following suggestions will be of help when such a situation arises.

But first a word of caution! When a diabetic first becomes ill, either he or some member of the family should get in touch with the doctor immediately. No changes should be made in the medical routine (insulin or tablets) or the dietary pattern without the doctor's permission. His instructions should be carefully followed.

These instructions may require that the three meals may have to be broken down into six or more feedings.

Included on the following pages are foods from the different exchange lists which are readily adaptable to liquid and soft diets. In addition you will find a number of recipes.

Milk Exchange List 1:

Milk is allowed in the diabetic diet in a stated amount. However, the milk allowance may be used in a variety of ways.

Milk may be served plain, either cold or hot as a beverage, or it may be served in combination with other foods such as egg-nogs, soups, gruel, etc. Recipes including milk will be found in the last section of this chapter.

127

For Vegetable Exchange List 2B, you might use —
2/3 cup tomato juice
or 2/3 cup mixed vegetable juice
or one of the following soups: 1. Chicken Rice Soup
2. Canned Condensed Soups
See recipes which follow in this chapter and soup recipes in chapter on Soups.

For one Fruit Exchange List 3, use one of the following (unsweetened):
1/3 cup apple juice
or ½ cup orange juice
or ½ cup grapefruit juice
or ¼ cup grape juice
or 1/3 cup pineapple juice
or ¼ cup prune juice
or 1/6 pint brick plain vanilla, chocolate, or strawberry ice cream. (Take off 1 Fat Exchange.)

Note: Dietetic or artificially sweetened ginger ale may be used without counting and may be mixed with any of the above juices without changing the food value. Grape juice and ginger ale are particularly good mixed together.

Bread Exchange List 4
For one Bread Exchange you may use one of the following:
cooked cereal — ½ cup
or prepared cereals — ¾ cup flaked
1 cup puffed
or 3 arrowroot crackers
or 4 social tea crackers
or 4 graham wafers
or 1 slice enriched white bread, plain or toasted.
or you may use 1½ Fruit Exchanges from List 3 in place of 1 Bread Exchange.

For instance, if you were using orange juice for the Bread Exchange, you would work out the amount as follows:
½ cup orange juice is one Fruit Exchange, therefore, ¾ cup orange juice would be 1½ Fruit Exchanges or the equivalent in food value of one Bread Exchange.

Meat Exchange List 5

In the acute stage of illness, foods from the Meat Exchange List may pose a problem. In such a case your doctor should be consulted about the best routine for you to follow under the circumstances. His instructions should be carefully followed.

Eggs may be used in eggnogs or custards.

One 3½ ounce can of pureed 'baby' meat may be exchanged for: 3 Meat Exchanges.

Fat Exchange List 6

Frequently in the acute stage of illness, fat is not well tolerated. This is often the case if the person is nauseated. Again, the doctor will advise the best procedure to follow.

Cream may be added to beverages such as tea, coffee, or cocoa. It may be used in the preparation of soft desserts or served with the desserts.

When Fluids are Important

When fever is present, the doctor may wish the patient to increase his fluid intake—and this is when the liquid low carbohydrate foods come into their own.

Some of these are:

1. Clear Broth: chicken, beef, etc., from which all the fat has been removed.
2. Consomme
3. Bouillon (canned or cubes)
4. Meat extract concentrates (diluted with water)
5. Artificially sweetened carbonated beverages available in liquid or tablet form, and in a variety of flavors.
6. Water
7. Clear Tea or Coffee

Vegetable Exchange List 2A

Tomato Juice 1/3 cup

Mixed Vegetable Juice 1/3 cup

CHICKEN RICE SOUP (Home-made)

Yield: 1 serving

Exchange for: 1 Foods used freely
and 1 Vegetable Exchange List 2B

Ingredients: 2/3 cup clear fat-free chicken broth, seasoned to taste
3 level tbsps. cooked rice

Method: Heat broth and rice together to desired serving temperature.

Variations with the same exchange value:

Chicken Noodle — use 3 tbsps. cooked noodles in place of the rice.

Beef Rice or Beef Noodle — make as above but use clear beef broth instead of chicken broth.

Beef with Barley — make as above and add 2 tbsps. cooked barley.

CANNED CONDENSED SOUPS

Yield: 1 serving

Exchange for: 1 Vegetable Exchange List 2B, and if milk is used for liquid, ½ Milk Exchange

Ingredients: 3 level tbsps. canned condensed soup
2/3 cup water, consomme, or clear fat-free broth
or ½ cup milk

Method: Mix above ingredients together and heat.

GRUEL

Yield: 1 serving

Exchange for: ½ Bread Exchange
and ½ Milk Exchange

Ingredients: ¼ cup cooked cereal
½ cup milk
artificial liquid sweetener to taste if desired
few grains ground nutmeg or ground cinnamon

Method: 1. Add hot milk to the hot cereal.
2. Mix very well so that there are no lumps.
3. Add artificial liquid sweetener.
4. Reheat. Sprinkle with cinnamon or nutmeg if desired. Serve hot.

BREAD AND MILK

Yield: 1 serving
Exchange for: 1 Bread Exchange
and ½ Milk Exchange
and 1 Fat Exchange
Ingredients: 1 slice bread
1 tsp. butter or margarine
½ cup milk
Method: 1. Butter bread with 1 tsp. butter or margarine.
2. Cut into cubes and place in cereal bowl.
3. Heat milk and pour over the bread cubes. Serve hot.

OMELET

Yield: 1 serving
Exchange for: 2 Meat Exchanges
and 1 Fat Exchange
Ingredients: 2 eggs, separated
pinch of baking powder
1 tbsp. water
salt and pepper to taste
1 tsp. butter or margarine
Method: 1. Beat egg whites until stiff; add baking powder.
2. Beat egg yolks until light; add salt and water, and beat slightly.
3. Heat an omelet pan and put in butter or margarine; have sides and bottom of pan well buttered.
4. Cut and fold egg whites into the egg yolk mixture.
5. Have pan very hot; pour in the egg mixture; spread evenly; reduce heat.
6. Cook slowly until omelet is set; place in moderate oven (350°F) to dry slightly on top.
7. Remove from oven, fold, and turn out; garnish and serve at once.

FRUIT NOG

Yield: 1 serving
Exchange for: 1 Meat Exchange
and 1 Fruit Exchange
Ingredients: 1 egg
½ cup orange juice or other fruit juice to the equivalent of 1 Fruit Exchange
Method: 1. Beat egg.
2. Add fruit juice and mix well; serve ice cold.

EGG NOG

Yield: 1 serving

Exchange for: 1 Meat Exchange
and ½ Milk Exchange

Ingredients: 1 egg
½ cup milk
artificial liquid sweetener to taste
1 or 2 drops vanilla

Method: 1. Beat egg and artificial liquid sweetener together.
2. Add milk and beat together until mixed, but not frothy.
3. Add vanilla; serve ice cold.

LEMONADE

Yield: 1 serving

Exchange for: 1 Foods used freely

Ingredients: 1 tbsp. lemon juice or 1 tbsp. unsweetened canned or frozen
lemon juice
½ tsp. or less artificial liquid sweetener
water
ice cubes

Method: Mix above ingredients together, adding ice cubes last.

HOT LEMONADE

Make as cold lemonade, omitting the ice cubes and adding hot water
instead of cold. Exchange as for cold lemonade.

GRAPE JUICE AND GINGER ALE

Yield: 1 serving

Exchange for: 1 Fruit Exchange
and 1 Foods as desired

Ingredients: ¼ cup unsweetened grape juice
artificially sweetened ginger ale
ice cubes if desired

Method: 1. Place grape juice in a glass.
2. Fill glass with ginger ale and mix.
3. Add ice if desired and serve.

Variations: The other fruit juices may also be mixed with artificially
sweetened ginger ale without adding to their food value.

LIMEADE

Yield: 1 serving

Exchange for: 1 Foods used freely

Ingredients: 1 tbsp. lime juice, fresh, canned, or frozen, without sugar
$\frac{1}{2}$ tsp. or less artificial liquid sweetener
water
ice cubes

Method: Mix above ingredients together, adding the ice cubes last.

ORANGE AND PINEAPPLE DRINK

Yield: 1 serving

Exchange for: 2 Fruit Exchanges

Ingredients: $\frac{1}{2}$ cup orange juice
1/3 cup pineapple juice
ice cubes if desired

Method: 1. Mix fruit juices together.
2. Add ice cubes or chopped ice. Serve.

OTHER SUGGESTIONS FOR LIQUID AND SOFT DIETS

1. Artificially sweetened applesauce, $\frac{1}{2}$ cup equals 1 Fruit Exchange.

2. Baked Custard — see page 95.

3. Lime Fluff — see page 100.

4. Flavored artificially sweetened jellies—Foods as desired.

5. Ice Cream — 1/6 pint brick ice cream or one ice cream roll may be exchanged for 1 Fruit Exchange and 1 Fat Exchange.

6. Ice Cream Jelly Bavarian — see page 105.

7. Rice Pudding — see page 97.

8. Soft Custard and other soft desserts from the dessert section — see page 95.

9. Coddled or poached egg.

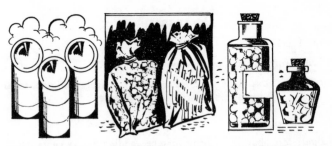

CANNING, FREEZING, PICKLING

For those who have the facilities, home preservation of fruits and vegetables at the peak of their season is an economical way of adding variety to the menu.

You CAN Can Without Sugar!

The keeping quality of canned fruit does not depend on the addition of sugar, but rather on sufficient processing and the use of sterile, airtight containers.

Some fruit mays lose a little color and flavor, but with care can be preserved to make an attractive product.

Special chemical preservatives are not necessary. Artificial sweeteners are best added after the fruit is opened for use, rather than being processed with the food.

Bulletins covering thoroughly the general directions for canning and freezing, etc., have sections on the preservation of food without sugar. For single copies write to your local Extension Service office or to the

U.S. Department of Agriculture
Washington, D.C.

Those persons on restricted sodium diets are reminded that the step in the prevention of discoloration called a "brine bath" used for certain fruits, must be avoided. But satisfactory results can be obtained by putting the fruit into acidulated water instead of brine bath. The acid to use could be vinegar or lemon juice — just sufficient to retain color of the fruit.

CANNING

The Hot Pack Method (or Boiling Water Bath) is the method most generally used for fruits and tomatoes. Do not attempt to can vegetables other than tomatoes and peppers unless you have a pressure cooker or a canner. These are especially designed to heat foods to higher temperatures than can be reached in the boiling water bath or steamer. The high temperature kills the harmful bacteria in non-acid food which may not be destroyed at boiling water temperature. The equipment required for hot pack method of preserving fruits is found in most homes and this is the method generally considered to be the safest and simplest for canning without sugar. A brief outline of this method follows, but for more detail, consult the bulletins mentioned. For canning with a pressure cooker, follow the directions of the manufacturer.

Hot Pack Method (Boiling Water Bath)

A large kettle, pail or wash boiler with closely fitting cover should be used. It should be fitted with a rack which allows circulation of water under the sealers. The canner should be deep enough to allow the water to cover the containers by at least two inches. If the water does not cover the containers, the food will not cook evenly.

Small Utensils

Essential tools include: sharp knives, a colander, bowls, measuring cups and spoons, towels, pie plates, wooden spoons, sauce pan to boil utensils. Jar lifters, wide-mouth funnel, strawberry huller, cherry-pitter, small brush, wire basket, cheese cloth, and cooking timers are also helpful.

Sealers (Jars)

Pint sealers or jars are easier to process and handle than larger sealers. There are two popular types. The screw top sealer with glass lid, rubber ring, and metal screw band, and the vacuum-type sealer with metal lid, edge lined with sealing compound, metal screw band or clamp.

Carefully check the sealers for cracks or chips. Check the lids. Use good metal rings. Use new rubber bands. The metal lids for the vacuum-type sealers cannot be used the second time.

Wash sealers and glass lids thoroughly and rinse. To sterilize, half fill the sealers with water and stand on a rack in a large kettle or boiler containing sufficient water to come half way up the sealers. Bring water to boiling point and leave sealers in the water until ready to fill. If using glass tops, they can be placed on the sealers while they are being sterilized. Rubber rings and metal lids should be dipped into boiling water before being placed on the sealers.

General Method:

1. Have all equipment ready.
2. Check and sterilize jars.
3. Boil small equipment you will use in the actual filling of the jars.
4. Use only firm fresh fruit. Wash carefully. Blanch.

To Blanch Fruit:

Tie fruit in square of cheesecloth or thin muslin, or place in colander. Plunge the fruit and colander or cloth into boiling water for 15 to 60 seconds. You should have three to four times as much water as fruit.

Reasons for Blanching:

To make removal of skins easier (tomatoes or peaches).

To shrink fruit so more can be packed into the jars.

To set color.

5. Cold Dip. Take quickly from the hot water and dip into cold water. Plunge it once or twice, but do not let it sit in the water any longer than necessary.
6. Slip off the skins or peel and pack fruit immediately into hot jars which have been sterilized. Do not let the jars cool.
7. Pour boiling water over the fruit in the jars, filling up to $\frac{1}{2}''$ from the top. Be sure there is no fruit above the level of the water.
8. Run a sterilized knife around in the jars to let out the air bubbles.
9. Put on the rubber rings which have been dipped into boiling water.
10. If using vacuum-type jars, seal the jars tightly at this point.
11. If using glass top jars, screw metal band tightly. Then loosen slightly, unscrewing not more than 1 inch.
12. Place filled sealers on rack 1'' apart in the boiling water bath. Have the water 2'' above the tops of the jars. Do not pour boiling water directly on sealers as jars might crack.
13. Place cover on bath, and bring to boiling point.
14. Start to count processing time from moment water is actually **Boiling Vigorously,** not just beginning to show bubbles. Keep water boiling until processing is finished, adding water if necessary to keep level 2'' above jars.
15. See table below for the processing times for the various fruits.
16. When processing time is up, immediately remove sealers from water to prevent overcooking. Place on folded dry cloth or newspapers.

To avoid cracking, do not place hot sealers in draughts or on metal or porcelain surfaces.

17. As soon as all bubbling in sealers has ceased, tighten tops on screw-top glass top sealers by giving the metal bands a final turn. Vacuum-type sealers require no further tightening since the seal is formed as they cool.

18. Cool sealers in an upright position, out of draughts. Leave space between sealers when cooling.

Test for Seal

Screw top jars: When cold, carefully invert each one for a minute or two, to see if there is leakage.

Vacuum type sealers with metal lids: when cold, gently tap lids with a spoon. If properly sealed, they will give a clear ringing note, and be curved slightly inwards. It is not necessary to invert vacuum-type sealers to test for seal.

FRUIT PROCESSING TABLE

Fruits	Preparation	Boiling Water	Time of Processing
Blueberries	Wash, clean, and pack in jars.	Fill jars with boiling water to ½″ of top.	16 min.
Dewberries Raspberries Strawberries Cherries Apricots Peaches Plums	Blanch by dipping in boiling water once or twice.	as above	16 min.
Rhubarb	Blanch as above, and cut in ½″ lengths.	as above	16 min.
Apples Pears Quinces Pineapple	Peel, core, cut in halves or slices.	as above	20 min.

APPLE CATSUP

Yield: Four ½ pint jars

Exchange 2 tsps. for: 1 Foods as desired

Ingredients: 4 cups cooked apples, sieved
2 tbsps. artificial liquid sweetener
1 tsp. ground cloves
1 tsp. dry mustard
1 tsp. cinnamon
1 tbsp. salt
2 onions
2 cups vinegar

Method: 1. Combine all ingredients except liquid sweetener. Mix well.
2. Bring to a boil. Simmer one hour.
3. Add liquid sweetener. While boiling hot, fill sterilized jars.
4. Seal tightly.

DILL PICKLES

Yield: 10-12 whole pickles

Exchange 1 pickle for: 1 Foods as desired

Method: Use freshly picked cucumbers, 3 to 5 inches long. Wash, soak overnight in cold water. Drain thoroughly. Place pieces of dill in bottom of clean jars. Pack cucumbers into jars and place more dill on top.

Combine: ½ cup table salt, or ¾ cup coarse salt, preferably not iodized
2 cups white vinegar
6 cups water

Bring to a boil and pour hot liquid over cucumbers. Seal. Let stand in a cool place at least 6 weeks before using.

ARTIFICIALLY SWEETENED GHERKINS OR MIXED PICKLES

Exchange: 4 pieces pickle for 1 Foods as desired

Most favorite pickle recipes can be followed, omitting the sugar and adding artificial liquid sweetener to taste Always add the artificial liquid sweetener near end of cooking time.

UNCOOKED TOMATO PICKLE

Yield: 5 pints

Exchange: The caloric value of this pickle is so low that it may be eaten in moderation as desired.

Ingredients: 4 quarts tomatoes
1½ cups chopped onion
¼ cup sweet red pepper, chopped
4 cups diced celery
2½ cups cider vinegar
½ cup salt
2 tbsps. mustard seed
artificial liquid sweetener to taste

Method:
1. Chop onion and tomatoes fine. Place in separate containers.
2. Add ¼ cup salt to each and let stand 3 hours. Mix tomato and onion; drain overnight.
3. Add remaining ingredients and pack in sterilized jars.

CHILI SAUCE

Yield: about six ½ pint jars

Exchange: The caloric value of this pickle is so low that it may be eaten in moderation as desired.

Ingredients: 18 tomatoes
2 green peppers
2 onions, medium
3 tbsps. artificial liquid sweetener
1 tbsp. salt
½ tsp. ground cloves
1 tsp. allspice
2 cups vinegar

Method:
1. Peel and chop tomatoes.
2. Chop peppers and onions fine.
3. Combine all ingredients **except** artificial liquid sweetener.
4. Boil slowly for four hours, or until sauce reaches desired thickness.
5. Add artificial liquid sweetener.
6. Pour boiling hot into sterilized jars. Seal.

Note: To make a brighter red sauce, use stick cinnamon, whole cloves, and whole allspice. Tie spices loosely in a piece of cheesecloth, and remove after cooking.

FRANKFURTER RELISH

Yield: about six ½ pint jars
Exchange 2 tsps. for: 1 Foods as desired
Ingredients: 3½ sweet red peppers
3 lbs. green peppers
3 lbs. onions
4 cups vinegar
1 tbsp. artificial liquid sweetener
1 tsp. mustard seed
1 tbsp. dry mustard
1 tbsp. celery seed
2 tbsps. salt

Method:
1. Wash peppers, remove cores and seeds.
2. Peel onions. Put onions and peppers through the food chopper, using medium knife blade. Cover with boiling water, and let stand 5 minutes.
3. Drain. Add vinegar, spices, and salt.
4. Cook until vegetables are tender (about 15 minutes) stirring occasionally.
5. Add artificial liquid sweetener. Pour boiling hot into sterilized jars. Seal.

SUGARLESS APRICOT MARMALADE

Exchange 2 tsps. for: 1 Foods as desired
Ingredients: 5 lbs. fresh apricots
1 lemon, diced
1 tbsp. artificial liquid sweetener (or more if desired)
½ pkg. powdered pectin
1 medium-sized orange, diced
1 cup pineapple, diced
3 tbsps. glycerin
dash of salt

Method:
1. Place chopped, cleaned apricots and other fruits in a kettle.
2. Simmer over low heat until fruit is soft (15 mins.)
3. Add powdered pectin and glycerin.
4. Bring to full rolling boil, and boil 1 minute.
5. Remove from heat and add artificial liquid sweetener.
6. Put into sterilized jars.
7. Process in boiling water for 30 minutes.
8. Follow directions for boiling water bath on previous pages.
9. Store in cool place (preferably in the refrigerator).

SUGARLESS GRAPE CONSERVE

Exchange 2 tsps. for: 1 Foods as desired

Ingredients: 5 lbs. grapes (concord)
grated orange rind from orange used for pulp
½ pkg. powdered pectin
1 cup diced orange pulp
4 tbsps. glycerin
2 tbsps. artificial liquid sweetener

Method: 1. Separate pulp from skins of grapes.
2. Bring pulp to boil in own juice.
3. Cover and simmer until easily separated from seeds. Strain.
4. Combine strained pulp with skins, and the orange rind.
5. Add powdered pectin and glycerin, and bring to a full rolling boil for 1 minute. (Hard boil that cannot be stirred down.) Add artificial liquid sweetener.
6. Place in sterilized jars.
7. Process in boiling water for 30 minutes. Follow directions for boiling water bath on previous page.
8. Store in a cool place (preferably in refrigerator.)

SIX FOOD EXCHANGE LISTS
for variety in meal planning

THIS IS NOT A DIET. The physician will prescribe the *amounts* or *number* of each of the exchanges which may be allowed each day.

Foods used freely

The following seasonings may be used freely, if desired:

Chopped parsley	Mint
Garlic	Onion
Celery	Nutmeg
Mustard	Cinnamon
Pepper and other spices	Saccharin
Lemon	Vinegar

Foods as desired

Some foods may be used as desired:

Rennet tablets
Pickles, sour
Pickles, unsweetened dill
Cranberries
Rhubarb

MILK EXCHANGES   LIST 1

One milk exchange contains:
Carbohydrate 12 grams, protein 8 grams, fat 10 grams: 170 calories

Amount to Use

Whole milk (plain or homogenized) .... 1 cup
*Skim milk .... 1 cup
Evaporated milk ....½ cup
Powdered whole milk ....¼ cup
*Powdered skim milk (non-fat dried milk) ....¼ cup
Buttermilk (made from whole milk) .... 1 cup
*Buttermilk (made from skim milk) .... 1 cup

*Skim milk products contain less fat. When exchanged for whole milk add
two fat exchanges to get the same food value.

VEGETABLE EXCHANGES   LIST 2

VEGETABLE EXCHANGES A contain: Negligible amounts of carbohydrate, protein, and fat. In raw form, size of serving unlimited; cooked, size serving ½ to 1 cup.

Asparagus
*Broccoli
Brussels sprouts
Cabbage
Cauliflower
Celery
*Chicory
Cucumber
*Escarole
Eggplant
Lettuce
Mushrooms
Okra
*Pepper
Radishes

*GREENS
    Beet greens
    Chard
    Collards
    Dandelion
    Kale
    Mustard
    Spinach
    Turnip greens
Sauerkraut
String beans, young
Summer squash
*Tomatoes per serving
*Watercress

VEGETABLE EXCHANGES B contain: Carbohydrate 7 grams, protein 2 grams: 35 calories. One serving equals ½ cup.

Beets
*Carrots
Onions
Peas, green

Pumpkin
Rutabagas
*Squash, winter
Turnips

*Contains considerable amount of vitamin A.

FRUIT EXCHANGES   LIST 3

One fruit exchange contains: Carbohydrate 10 grams: 40 calories. Fruits may be fresh, dried, cooked, canned or frozen as long as no sugar is added.

Amount to Use

Apple (2″ dia.)	1 small
Applesauce	½ cup
Apricots, fresh	2 medium
Apricots, dried	4 halves
Banana	½ small
Blackberries	1 cup
Raspberries	1 cup
*Strawberries	1 cup
Blueberries	⅔ cup
*Cantaloupe (6″ dia.)	¼
Cherries	10 large
Dates	2
Figs, fresh	2 large
Figs, dried	1 small
*Grapefruit	½ small
*Grapefruit juice	½ cup
Grapes	12
Grape juice	¼ cup
Honeydew melon, medium	⅛
Mango	½ small
*Orange	1 small
*Orange juice	½ cup
Papaya	⅓ medium
Peach	1 medium
Pear	1 small
Pineapple	½ cup
Pineapple juice	⅓ cup
Plums	2 medium
Prunes, dried	2 medium
Raisins	2 tablespoons
*Tangerine	1 large
Watermelon	1 cup

*Contains considerable amount of vitamin C (ascorbic acid).

147

BREAD EXCHANGES LIST 4

One bread exchange contains: Carbohydrate 15 grams, protein 2 grams: 70 Calories.

Amount to Use

Bread	1 slice
Biscuit, roll (2" dia.)	1
Muffin (2" dia.)	1
Cornbread (1½" cube)	1
Cereals, cooked	½ cup
Dry, flake & puff types	¾ cup
Rice, grits, cooked	½ cup
Spaghetti, noodles, cooked	½ cup
Macaroni, cooked	½ cup
Crackers, graham (2½" sq.)	2
Oysterettes (½ cup)	20
Saltines (2" sq.)	5
Soda (2½" sq.)	3
Round, thin	6
Flour	2½ tablespoons
Vegetables	
Beans and peas, dried, cooked	½ cup
(lima, navy, split peas, cowpea, etc.)	
Baked beans, no pork	¼ cup
Corn	⅓ cup
Popcorn	1 cup
Parsnips	⅔ cup
Potatoes, white	1 small
Potatoes, white, mashed	½ cup
Potatoes, sweet or yams	¼ cup
Sponge cake, plain (1½" cube)	1
Ice cream (omit two fat exchanges)	½ cup

MEAT EXCHANGES   LIST 5

One meat exchange contains: Protein 7 grams, fat 5 grams: 75 calories. An average size serving of meat would be 3 meat exchanges or two meat balls, a small steak, (¼ lb. raw weight) or three of any of the foods listed below.

Amount to Use

Meat and poultry (medium fat)...1 ounce
    (Beef, lamb, pork, liver, chicken, etc.)
Cold cuts (4½″ x ⅛″) ....1 slice
    Salami, minced ham, Bologna, Liverwurst, luncheon loaf
Frankfurter (8-9 per lb.)...1
Egg 1
Fish: haddock, flounder, bass, etc...1 ounce
    Salmon, tuna, crab, lobster ....¼ cup
    Shrimp, clams, oysters, etc. ....5 small
    Sardines ....3 medium
Cheese, Cheddar type ....1 ounce
    cottage ....¼ cup
Peanut butter ....2 tablespoons

FAT EXCHANGES   LIST 6

One fat exchange contains: Fat 5 grams: 45 calories.

Amount to Use

Butter or margarine	1 teaspoon
Bacon, crisp	1 slice
Cream, light	2 tablespoons
Cream, heavy	1 tablespoon
Cream cheese	1 tablespoon
Avocado (4″ diameter)	⅛
French dressing	1 tablespoon
Mayonnaise	1 teaspoon
Oil or cooking fat	1 teaspoon
Nuts	6 small
Olives	5 small

NOTES

NOTES